The VACCINE
NARRATIVE

The VACCINE NARRATIVE

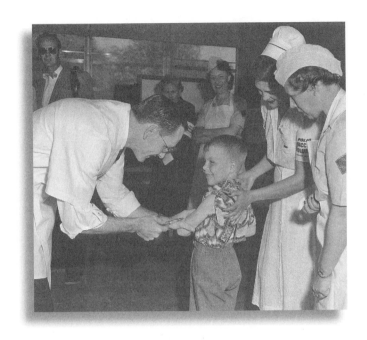

Jacob Heller

VANDERBILT UNIVERSITY PRESS

NASHVILLE

12   11   10   09   08   1   2   3   4   5

This book is printed on acid-free paper.
Manufactured in the United States of America

Designed by Cheryl Carrington

Frontispiece: Randy Kerr receives the first polio
vaccination in field trial, McLean, VA, April 26, 1954.
Courtesy of March of Dimes Birth Defects Foundation.

Library of Congress Cataloging-in-Publication Data

Heller, Jacob, Ph.D.
The vaccine narrative / Jacob Heller. — 1st ed.
p.   ; cm.
Includes bibliographical references and index.
ISBN 978-0-8265-1590-2 (cloth : alk. paper)
ISBN 978-0-8265-1591-9 (pbk. : alk. paper)
1. Vaccines—History.   2. Vaccines—Social aspects.
3. Vaccines—Historiography.   I. Title.
[DNLM: 1. Vaccines—history—United States.
2. Communicable Disease Control—history—United
States. 3. History, 20th Century—United States.
4. Sociology, Medical—United States.
5. Vaccination—history—United States.
QW 11 AA1 H477v 2008]
RA638.H45 2008
615'.372—dc22
2007022442

Contents

Acknowledgments

This book began as an idea shared in a research workshop at Stony Brook University with Mandy Frisken, Lisa Handler, Anna Linders, and Diane Samuels. Since then, it has undergone numerous incarnations.

Bob Zussman, Nancy Tomes, Ian Roxborough, and Naomi Rosenthal have been crucial to the foundations of the book. Special thanks go to Bob, who has never hesitated to tell me when things did not look, sound, or read well, for which I thank him sincerely—he helped make this book much better than it would otherwise be. My editor at Vanderbilt, Michael Ames, has managed to be encouraging and supportive while keeping me clear about the priorities in producing a book like this one. His availability, advice, and no-nonsense attitude have made this last step in the process both pleasant and rewarding, as have the entire staff at Vanderbilt University Press. James Colgrove and the anonymous reviewer gave me insightful and challenging comments on the manuscript. I want to thank all my colleagues in the Sociology Department at SUNY College at Old Westbury for their general collegiality and support, but special thanks goes to Gilda Zwerman for her support, comments, and attitude.

My deepest debt remains to my best friend and fellow traveler, who long advised me to consider this a book (rather than a series of articles), and who has amazingly manifested faith in both me and the project. She is, was, and remains my best reader, editor, and critic.

The VACCINE NARRATIVE

Introduction

▰ Vaccines in Context

Vaccines have been part of Western medicine and public health for more than two hundred years. They have become more than just a way to stay healthy: they have become a metaphor for protection and a cultural story

> ✕ *The vaccine was a folk victory, an occasion for pride and jubilation.*
>
> —Richard Carter
> *Breakthrough: The Saga of Jonas Salk*

that transcends social divides. We simultaneously understand vaccines as a shield against disease, a right of passage for children and parents, and an expression of our science, civilization, modernity, and morality. We want to make sure our children get all the necessary "shots" to grow up healthy and to have a fair chance at life's opportunities; we want children throughout the world to benefit from this simple, elegant intervention that eradicates unnecessary suffering. Vaccines have taken on important meanings far beyond the realm of medicine and public health.

New vaccines still manage to excite our imagination and allay our fears about disease, even though controversies sometimes develop about their use, their cost, and their consequences. Pharmaceutical giant Merck & Co. recently came out with two new vaccines: one against human papilloma virus (HPV), to prevent and eventually eradicate cervical cancer (Blumenthal 2007), and another that promises protection against rotavirus, a debilitating and potentially deadly diarrhea-causing infection among children, particularly the poorest of the poor (Harris 2006). Both have been certified as highly effective, but both have also raised issues of cost, access, the nature of the target population, and whether these vaccines are necessary and appropriate for the American population. Recent scientific discoveries and sizable investments promise further vaccine triumphs: against the much-feared but still uncertain avian flu pandemic (Davis 2005), against HIV/AIDS (Altman 2006), or even against smoking

(Tuller 2006). With a stable of established vaccines and promising new ones in development, vaccines appear to be simple and versatile tools for contending with all kinds of as-yet-unforeseen problems. As new diseases arise, we have faith that scientists will study the problem, develop and test vaccines that, with widespread use, will protect us, and put the new diseases on the road to extinction.

Every vaccine has costs and benefits that sometimes seem unfair. Health professionals and women's health advocates have, for example, raised concerns about the target population for the new HPV vaccine and how to achieve high levels of compliance with recommended use. Since most girls and women only contract HPV from boys and men, some women's health advocates have asked why the vaccine has not been designed to target the entire HPV-carrying population—boys as well as girls, men as well as young women. Moreover, widespread use of Pap smears has already drastically reduced the consequences of HPV infection for American women, and this has raised questions about whether Americans really need an HPV vaccine at all (Rabin 2006). Others have raised questions about mandating a vaccine to protect young women from a sexually transmitted virus (Daitz 2006; Uribarri 2007).

Public and heated controversies like those surrounding HPV vaccine, however, rarely concern the vaccine itself, which typically receives high and hopeful praise once it has passed scientific muster.[1] Instead, conflicts seem to arise around the context: the laws regarding vaccine use, the role of corporate lobbying, or the politics of a vaccine designed to protect against a controversial disease. There is also the cost issue. We understand vaccines as such a good bargain for society as a whole that out-of-pocket costs to vaccine recipients often become a side issue: our belief in the efficacy, necessity, and wisdom of vaccines sometimes overrides more mundane aspects like the price at the point of use. Yet the cumulative costs of the full course of vaccines for children, none of which is free, has made a surprising number of doctors reluctant to administer them (Pollack 2007). Understanding these changes, tracing them over time, and imagining what the future may hold for vaccines is not, however, as straightforward as the vaccines themselves seem to be. Individual vaccines or diseases may not change much from year to year or even decade to decade, but their context undergoes slow and continuous variation that subtly influences how we view, understand, and use vaccines.

Since Edward Jenner discovered the first vaccine (against smallpox) in the 1790s, vaccines have enjoyed a widely varied career in America. The current faith in vaccines was not always so widespread, which raises the question of how our strong cultural acceptance of vaccines came about. Today, vaccines are highly respected and compliance rates hover near all-time highs, despite a steady decline in attitudes towards the health care system. Americans have become increasingly skeptical about the motives and outcomes associated with modern medicine (CDC 2003; Schlesinger 2002). How have vaccines withstood this general trend? As we consider more vaccines for children (the typical American child will receive more than twenty shots by school age, not including the new HPV or rotavirus vaccines), the high cost of vaccine development, and the controversies that vaccines can create, it becomes imperative to explore not just the origins of specific vaccines, but how we have come to understand and respect them. Something in our common past has put vaccines in a different class than the medical profession, hospitals, or other medical or public health measures; acceptance of vaccines is widespread, normative, and persistent over time. What explains our continuing faith in vaccines, particularly in the face of those rare vaccines that not only disappoint, but perhaps cause harm?

A full and valid understanding about vaccines depends on knowledge about their historical and cultural aspects, even more than knowledge about their efficacy or chemistry. It is, after all, possible for people to reject an effective and rational innovation. Analyzing vaccines' cultural foundations can help us contextualize current and future vaccine-related challenges—whether they concern a vaccine against HPV, HIV/AIDS, or some as-yet-unknown disease we will encounter in the future. Our historical experience of vaccines necessarily informs our present and future behaviors. Because not all events have equal impacts, the historical investigation of how we understand vaccines starts not at the chronological beginning, but with what is undoubtedly the most famous—and most familiar—vaccine story we know.

▮ Polio: A Familiar Story

Through the first half of the twentieth century, American children risked contracting polio any time they went outside during the summer. Following the massive polio epidemic in 1952, parents were particularly worried about the disease. As historian Jane Smith describes in her popular account of the discovery of the Salk polio vaccine,

> To the parents of the 1950s, there was nothing routine about polio. Everyone knew someone whose child had been stricken, who had gone to bed one day complaining of a headache and had never

walked again. Everyone saw them, the valiant toddler learning to lurch across the floor with his leg in a brace, the speed demon who had traded in his first bike for a wheelchair, the teenager who would never dance at her high school prom. (Smith 1990, 21–22)

Polio had become a worst-case scenario for an infectious disease. Without warning, it struck children and young people across social and economic lines with symptoms as benign as fever, sore throat, and headache that could lead to varying degrees of paralysis or even death. No one knew much about the disease, how it was transmitted, or why some people caught it and others did not. The only recourse for doctors was to use poorly understood leg braces and casts (which they found by 1940 to be implicated in paralysis), or the radical treatment devised by an Australian nun, Elizabeth Kenny, that involved physical therapy and the painful application of hot wet towels to the bodies of the afflicted (Rogers 1992). Many polio survivors were eventually enclosed in iron-lung machines whose only function was to keep the victims alive, but did not contribute to their cure; others were left with varying degrees of paralysis. Even the new wonder drugs, penicillin and its cousins, were useless against polio. No one could cure, predict, or prevent the disease.

In April of 1955, however, news spread that Dr. Jonas E. Salk had developed a vaccine that would reliably prevent paralytic polio. Driven by his own personal dedication and the unwavering support of the National Foundation for Infantile Paralysis (The March of Dimes), Salk had conducted the painstaking research, completed the elaborate and public trials, and discovered a vaccine that would save millions of American children from polio. The victory has been widely lauded: "More than a scientific achievement, the vaccine was a folk victory, an occasion for pride and jubilation. A contagion of love swept the world" (Carter 1966, 1). People were jubilant, and understandably so. The constant fear under which Americans had lived for two generations lifted from their lives in one grand moment. Medical science had fulfilled its promise: it had found a vaccine and was about to vanquish polio.

With Salk's polio vaccine, killed polio germs mobilized the body's own natural defenses to protect each individual from infection and disease, and through these individuals the entire population. Immunity from polio was the gift that Salk and the vaccine offered Americans. Salk seemed to understand the scope and grandeur of his contribution when in answer to the question from Edward R. Murrow, "Who owns the patent on this vaccine?" he responded, "Well, the people, I would say. There is no patent. Could you patent the sun?" (Murrow and Salk 1955).

Authors, biographers, journalists, children's authors, and encyclopedists have told and retold the polio story, and hailed it as a breakthrough. It is a story of success against the odds: how the rational and systematic application of science in the hands of a dedicated scientist—a humble genius (Salk)—defeated the disease and prevented its horribly crippling effects, including its ultimate consequence, death. It is the story of how science taught the human body to marshal its defenses to protect against polio (Martin 1994). It substantiates and reinforces Americans' belief in the process and institutions of medical discovery that protect their health; American medical science fights deadly disease—and wins.

Of course, the history of polio and polio vaccines is far more complex than this condensed outline suggests, and researchers have painstakingly detailed the account of the long, difficult struggle that culminated in the Salk vaccine (Carter 1966; Paul 1971; Klein 1972; Brandt 1978; Smith 1990). Salk's breakthrough had been preceded by decades of failed efforts by him and other researchers (Dowling 1977). But we know this: we know that polio vaccine saved thousands from paralysis and death, and despite difficulties, polio rates have fallen to zero—with no cases of wild polio in North or South America since 1991 (Pickering 2000). The system worked, and the story of polio vaccine remains the story of the conquest of a terrible disease.

Narratives in Action— Unpacking Polio's Story

The case of polio vaccine in the 1950s is almost certainly the best-known vaccination story in American history.[2] It is central to Americans' cultural understanding of vaccines; it has become both the archetype and an instantiation of modern vaccination. It crowds together contrasting images: on the one hand, crippled children remain trapped in metal braces or doomed to live in iron-lung machines while on the other, happily vaccinated children run and play without fear. The contrast is so stark, and the putative intervention so small and innocuous, that the conclusion seems unavoidable: vaccines are cheap, safe, and effective; they rescue us from dreaded infectious disease. Polio was a serious and terrifying disease. Salk's research and vaccine were lifesaving breakthroughs. The polio case elevates scientific discovery to the level of a cultural narrative.

In reality, most polio cases fell into the category called "minor illness of poliomyelitis" and were entirely without symptoms, and many others led to only low-grade fevers without any serious consequences (Paul 1971). Fear of the much rarer neurological damage (paralysis), together with active anti-polio campaigning by the March of Dimes and the early involvement of Franklin Delano Roosevelt, the most famous polio sufferer, made polio, with its apparent randomness, appear far more frightening than other diseases that were sickening more people and causing many more deaths. Some have argued persuasively that at times the social construction of polio as a disease made it much more of a problem in the public's mind than objective morbidity and mortality rates could ever have done (Aronowitz 1992). Moreover, though the Salk trials were highly publicized and reported to be a great success, the vaccine cut the incidence of polio only in half compared to the control groups (Baker 2000)—hardly the dramatic preventive in which we have come to believe. Heightened fears about polio increased the impact of the Salk vaccine discovery. There were disappointments, as well.

The most famous Salk vaccine failure came early on, when a batch of vaccine manufactured by Cutter Pharmaceuticals used in the culminating 1955 clinical trials began to cause paralytic polio in children, instead of protecting them from it (e.g., Furman 1955). National concerns prompted an immediate federal investigation, and vaccine laboratory procedures were quickly changed and recertified as safe; the glitch had been overcome and vaccine production and mass vaccination of children resumed.

The Salk vaccine's less famous but more lasting failures were not related to bad batches, but to the very nature of his vaccine. The Salk vaccine was difficult to administer because it required two shots, which created logistical and administrative problems. Vaccines by themselves do not prevent disease, they need to be delivered to the susceptible population, usually as part of an effective vaccination campaign. Perhaps as importantly, researchers soon found that Salk's vaccine failed to produce lasting immunity. Within five years of the Salk vaccine debut, the FDA approved a second polio vaccine, this one made with attenuated (weakened) live cells, and administered in one oral dose. Developed by Albert Sabin, this version conferred years-long immunity, was easier to administer, and became for thirty-five years the American polio vaccine of choice, though not without its own safety controversies (Paul 1971). Does this mean that Salk was a fake, or that his vaccine had no promise? Far from it; since 1997, official experts began recommending an improved inactivated (killed) cell vaccine, modeled on Salk's original idea (Pickering 2000). But Salk's vaccine was nothing near the panacea we have come to know it to be: the Salk vaccine did not immediately solve the polio problem. Shortly after the introduction of the Salk vaccine, polio morbidity declined, but as late as 1961 its widespread administration was still referred to by March of Dimes head Basil O'Connor as a continuing massive "trial" (Paul 1971, 463). How, then, did Salk's vaccine get so much credit?

The Salk vaccine came at a very particular point in history. By the 1950s, medical institutions were approaching what would be the apex of their power and prestige (Starr 1982). In this pre-Sputnik postwar period, enthusiasm supported by economic growth and general prosperity seemed to suggest that there might, indeed, be no limit to the heights of accomplishment. Science had begun to promise that it would rid the world of starvation, disease, and other scourges. The ethic of American can-do-ism prepared people to expect successes just like Salk's, in which scientific and technological know-how accomplished the previously unthinkable. The Salk vaccine trials and the publicity that followed were a logical step in the fulfillment of those promises. The story we tell and retell about Salk and his vaccine remains one that embodies the spirit of heroism, altruism, and the smooth success of science and ingenuity. It is difficult to acknowledge contradictions of our shared knowledge about Salk, polio vaccine, and the good that they produced.

Perhaps polio vaccination has achieved its place in our collective sense of vaccines because of specific aspects of the polio case. The search for a polio vaccine was public, dramatic, and took place at a time when fear of polio was uppermost in many Americans' minds (though other diseases presented greater public health risks, for example tuberculosis, influenza, and many of the chronic diseases like cancer and heart disease). For polio, unlike some other diseases, there were few practical alternatives to a vaccine, and once the Salk vaccine gained acceptance, there seemed little reason for the public to worry about other options. After application of the Salk vaccine, polio rates fell, though the most dramatic decline[3] happened after widespread use of the Sabin vaccine. In hindsight, a vaccine seems the natural solution to the problem of epidemic polio.

We can catch only glimpses of the pervasive power of the polio story and its ability to guide what we see because—by its nature—a cultural narrative precludes contravening evidence. In the quotation from Jane Smith's book at the beginning of the previous section, the author asserts that "everyone knew someone" who had been stricken. This has become a commonplace of the polio story. On the following page of her book, she acknowledges, however, that, "unlike so many others, I had no direct contact with polio, no friends or relatives who were paralyzed" (Smith 1990, 23). What is interesting here is not the slip of the author's statements, but the ease with which the contradiction flows; Smith discounts the evidence of her own first-hand experience in favor of a cultural narrative. This is precisely the nature of a cultural narrative—an economical story that elides and overwhelms contradictions, and simplifies our understanding of reality with scripted meanings and metaphors so that we can more easily make sense of the whole. So: polio becomes a widespread and ever-present danger completely routed by Salk's unproblematic vaccine.

Given the polio vaccine story, it is hardly surprising that Americans invest such faith in vaccines. By the beginning of the twenty-first century and despite extremely low incidence of vaccine-preventable infectious disease in the United States, vaccine compliance rates for school-age children had reached all-time highs (CDC 2003). Both medical experts and lay people generally credit vaccines as our saviors from infectious disease and death. As one children's book about vaccines put it, "from the earliest bronze axes to the most recent computers, from dugout canoes to supersonic jets . . . probably none of these things has so profoundly aided humanity as the invention of vaccines" (Collier 2004, 9). Such assessments, however, remain bound up with the broader American cultural narrative of vaccines and vaccination. Coming at the halfway point in the twentieth century, Salk's polio vaccine served two important purposes for the reputation of vaccines, aside from any empirically verifiable public health benefits. The Salk vaccine story presented a neatened and clarified version to supplant more equivocal vaccine stories (most notably smallpox, rabies, and diphtheria, along with numerous "failed" vaccines), and it made vaccination a positive good.

Master Narratives and Vaccines

This book is about the social construction of meanings for vaccines in American culture. It analyzes four different vaccine cases spanning the twentieth century: diphtheria, rubella (German measles), pertussis (whooping cough), and HIV/AIDS.[4] Each case comes from an important period in the history of American medical and public health, and is, as a result, important in the evolution of cultural meaning for vaccines and vaccination. Out of these disparate cases, a coherent and robust vaccine "master narrative" emerges. A master narrative is an overarching storyline or sequence of events that anticipates and therefore reinforces our established expectations (Maines 1999). It is a culturally understood template for the stories we tell about aspects of our lives—in this case about vaccines and vaccination. Given that such a narrative exists, investigation into its nature and origins helps to understand not only vaccines as a cultural (as opposed to strictly medical or scientific) phenomenon, but also how such narratives can work in areas of life generally thought to be governed by more widely accepted explanations, like interest, power, and utility. A master narrative does not displace these kinds of explanations for how and why American culture has used vaccines (medical efficacy, cost/benefit risk calculations, institutional clout, industrial profit, etc.); it supplements those arguments with a new source of support that can be both powerful and flexible.

A master narrative is different than an ideology or a value system, or even an established set of practices and beliefs, though it can interact with all of these. Narratives always incorporate a specific sequence of events with particular consequences (Riessman 2004). The reliance on "story" makes a master narrative a different animal than more concrete phenomena, and subject to different kinds of rules. Stories provide enduring metaphors to frame and guide ideas, expectations, practices, and beliefs. But they do this without employing evidence or argument; narratives use *stories* to do their work. Polletta's work on the role of narratives in social movements found that the persuasive nature of stories often overwhelmed the facts surrounding events they sought to describe (Polletta 1998). The same seems to apply to vaccination—our stories guide our understanding of vaccines and vaccination in ways that can be, if not impervious, certainly highly resistant to facts, evidence, and argument. As Emily Martin (1994) found, Americans—including scientists—understand immunity in terms of metaphors.

We might expect an enthusiastic reception for vaccination during the height of a national panic about polio (or AIDS or another contagious and dangerous disease), but Americans accept vaccines and vaccination today without much danger from the diseases against which the vaccines offer protection. We have hardly any experiential basis for our relationship to vaccination; aside from AIDS, most people have little or no first-hand contact with deadly epidemic disease. Few Americans have the technical knowledge to understand the research findings that support vaccine use. Where do our ideas about vaccination come from? As with any practice that does not provide immediate benefits, gratification, results, or rescue, we need to believe in vaccines to accept their continued use.

The simple explanation for vaccines' continued public support is that vaccination works; the technical knowledge has been transformed into lay knowledge, something people can grasp without the baggage of scientific jargon and data. (This is also, in important ways, part of the narrative of vaccines: science works and deserves our trust.) Such an explanation begs the question of how acceptance reached current high levels. Its teleology confuses the fact that vaccines are widely accepted with evidence explaining wide acceptance. It mistakes the "container for the thing contained" (Thurber 1957, 53). The project here is to understand the relationship between research and the meanings that grew out of it, as well as the ways in which those meanings in turn influenced and guided the interpretation of subsequent research. How important are the stories about vaccination for the social construction of disease prevention and the cultural value of vaccines and vaccination? The strong correspondence between the way vaccines have been talked about within the health professions and in the general culture suggests that vaccines' metaphorical meanings, even for health professionals, have strong cultural currency.

Whether it is the story of the dramatic polio trials in the 1950s, the hopeful predictions for the banishment of AIDS, or the stories we tell children (and ourselves) when we take them to be vaccinated, the idea of a master narrative argues that those stories are thematically subsidiary to the dominant story of the culture's relationship to vaccines. As described below and in the succeeding chapters, these data show how the role of professional consensus and attitudes have been central to the construction of the vaccination narrative. Researchers' willingness to conduct their work within the narrative's boundaries has meant that its existence and underlying assumptions have been important for researchers—the profession of medicine or bacteriology does not carry an exemption from cultural influences—as well as for average Americans. In recognizing and understanding the development and workings of a vaccine master narrative, it is possible to appreciate the role of story and narrative in our lives and have a chance to see outside the narratives of specific vaccines for a better and clearer look at both the master narrative of vaccines and the vaccines themselves.

■ Elaborating the Vaccine Master Narrative

Like all cultural narratives, the vaccine narrative is not complicated, and it is rarely challenged. As the polio story tells us, vaccines consummate the thrifty American bargain: an ounce of prevention worth a pound of cure. Most of all, we take from the narrative the overarching idea that vaccines work. Vaccines receive credit for the substantial reductions in infectious disease in developed areas of the world (Parish 1965), even when they are being critiqued (e.g. Wilson 1967; Howson, Howe, and Fineberg 1991; Moore and Anderson 1994). Despite growing public disenchantment with physicians and recent medical institutions stemming in part from changing institutional contexts for the provision of health care (Jones 1981; Rothman and Rothman 1984; Rothman 1991; Schlesinger 2002), there is little public dissent from the idea that vaccination is an unequivocal good. Recent evidence of interesting patterns of vaccination compliance support the idea that vaccination has broad (if not perhaps deep) support among the general population (Smith, Chu, and Barker 2004).

Unlike changes in medical practice that can be implemented directly by physicians—which is not to say without contention or negotiation with patients or other non-physicians (e.g. Leavitt 1986)—vaccination is tied to public health and therefore to public policy. Vaccines promise to confer immunity to specific diseases in the vaccinated individual: a dose of measles vaccine promises to protect a child from contracting measles. But, except in special cases, the use of vaccines involves the protection of communities, not simply individuals, and so vaccines' primary use has been as part of mass vaccination programs. This employs the concept of *herd protection*, and holds that only a limited, statistically determined proportion of a population needs to possess individual immunity to a particular disease in order for the entire population to remain protected from the disease (Paul 2004). In New York State, to cite a typical example, anyone born after 1957 must show evidence of measles vaccination or immunity in order to attend college. This policy uses the logic of herd immunity to require all college students to show proof of measles vaccination to protect the population of college students as a whole. Any particular measles vaccine shot can be expected to have only limited efficacy (it protects, on average, only a percentage of the people who receive the measles shot), but the nature of herd protection is such that with sufficient coverage, even an imperfect vaccine can effectively immunize the community, though each individual may not be resistant to measles. The vaccination law applies to each individual in order to protect the larger community from epidemic measles. The idea of herd immunity implies that any student who refuses to be vaccinated, then, risks more than her own health—she puts at risk the larger community's ability to protect itself from an epidemic. This asks each individual to accept her own vaccination for the greater good.

The accounts of vaccines described in children's books are particularly revealing because they intentionally set out culturally normative values about vaccines; they aim to instruct. Here we find a crystallized version of the narrative. Despite the use of child-friendly words, it is the same explanation of vaccination we know in everyday life. A complicated immunological explanation that relies on probability, epidemiology, and herd immunity becomes a simple story of attack, defense, protection, and safety, with some biology vocabulary thrown in:

[S]cientists made a vaccine from measles virus that was carefully neutralized to do no harm. When the vaccine is given to children, their lymphocytes react as if the virus is still dangerous. The "measles squad" multiplies rapidly, making antibodies and killer cells. If the original measles virus attacks a child after he or she has been vaccinated, the lymphocyte measles squad "remembers" the virus in double-quick time. They defeat it before any damage is done. Vaccinated children are protected from measles for the rest of their lives. (Balkwill 2002, 29)

Vaccines "do no harm," they create "squads" that defeat invading attackers, leading to life-long protection. The story is simple and unequivocal; it talks about individual protection in reassuringly scientific terms.

Despite important differences between measles and rabies vaccines, the juvenile literature tells of the serendipitous discovery of rabies vaccine in strikingly similar terms:

Louis Pasteur . . . noticed that people who survived a dangerous disease, like rabies, were never troubled by it again. Pasteur's idea was to introduce a small amount of the disease into a person's body. His ultimate intention was to protect the person from a more serious attack. Pasteur did this to a young boy named Joseph Meister. Joseph had been bitten by a rabid dog. Pasteur injected Joseph with a small does of serum from a rabbit that had died of rabies. When Joseph survived the rabies attack, Pasteur realized his test had worked. The small dose of rabies had somehow protected Joseph from the more dangerous infection. (Almonte and Desmond 1991, 25)

The narrative appears consistent: a measured and safe "small dose" vaccine can protect us from disease. Yet in these two cases, the vaccine (treated as a monolithic protector) actually works differently. For measles, the vaccine prepares the body to defend against future attacks; this is called *active* immunity, because it stimulates the immune system to produce antibodies against a specific antigen (measles germs). Pasteur's rabies vaccine confers protection *after* the child, Joseph Meister, has already been bitten—his defenses must already be activated. This vaccine works because the rabbit serum contains the rabbit's antitoxin, a chemical that the rabbit produced to deal (unsuccessfully) with its own case of rabies, but which in Joseph Meister continues to confer enough temporary, *passive*, immunity for him to recover. Calling both vaccines elides these differences and merges both into the same narrative of protection from disease conferred by a "shot" that is neither a medicine nor a cure. The same pattern extends to the use of toxoids (weakened toxins, as against diphtheria), killed or attenuated vaccines (as for polio), therapeutic vaccines (for AIDS), and even contraceptive vaccines (Norplant)—regardless of differences, they all fall under the same rubric, and therefore serve as interchangeable vaccine players in their stories, which conform to the cultural narrative we have of vaccines.

Reporting about vaccines for an adult lay audience follows the same pattern. This excerpt from a 1947 front-page article in the *New York Times* followed two smallpox deaths in the Bronx:

> The Mayor said that . . . the only sure method of preventing the spread of smallpox in the city was to persuade every resident to submit to vaccination, which is not compulsory by law. At the mayor's request Dr. Rivers [of the Board of Health] summarized his view of the situation, "Smallpox cannot be prevented in any way except vaccination," he declared. "No quarantine or isolation will do it. Vaccination is the oldest and still one of the best methods, if not the best. The situation is not alarming, but it is disturbing. There have been two deaths and if preventive measures are delayed any longer the Mayor might be criticized both from within and without the city. What he urges is taking time by the forelock, not a stampede. It is just a case of taking sound measures to forestall an emergency." (NYT 1947)

The rationale New York's Mayor O'Dwyer endorsed is difficult to challenge; it lays out quite clearly the narrative expectation that though only two have died (a husband and wife), all are in danger and vaccination will protect the population. It expects all 7,800,000 New Yorkers to "submit to vaccination" because that is the only way they can protect themselves. The vaccine narrative, like all stories, contains a moral: vaccines are the best and only way to contend with infectious disease.

Nursing textbooks offer a different perspective on the narrative. The job in these books (with regard to vaccination) is to prepare health professionals to accomplish the greatest coverage for all vaccine preparations; if vaccination were a religion, these books would serve as part of the training for missionaries. Like the call by Dr. Rivers above, this quotation forsakes the herd theory of immunity, on which mass vaccination policies are based, in favor of complete coverage (irrespective of the specific vaccine).

> The thinking of health authorities in government is that immunization programs are effective only if all comply. Nurses have a clear responsibility to use their knowledge about immune processes and the processes of transmission to encourage people actively to take advantage of immunization programs within their community. (Ellis and Nowlis 1994, 367)

The epidemiological fact, however, is that not all need comply for the population to enjoy immunity. Moreover, by insisting on universal compliance, the injunction to achieve one hundred percent vaccine coverage turns the small portions of the population who do not comply (for whatever reasons) into deviants who need to be cajoled into full compliance with vaccine policies. This sets the stage for one of the necessary characters in any compelling narrative: the opponent.

Who are the people that oppose vaccination? The call on "knowledge" implicitly asserts that non-compliance with vaccination policies is a product of ignorance. The idea that ignorance and (by implication, irrational) fear are the main reasons for non-compliance with vaccination policies reinforces the nursing mission to overcome prejudice with knowledge (from science) and good practices. The emphasis on bringing the practical application of vaccination to bear on those segments of society that have not yet benefited from it stresses each nurse's role as a monitor of good practices. Compliance is a good unto itself, it would seem, and this value is so ingrained into the culture of modern American health professions that it can remain unspoken and still carry authority.

When the narrative is challenged, it sometimes gains strength. Throughout the history of vaccination, the response to opponents of vaccination has reasserted the narrative in terms designed not so much to refute specific negative claims about vaccines, as to undermine their applicability. Here, another nursing handbook prepares its readers to contend with arguments against vaccination. It classifies skepticism about vaccination as a product of fear and media attention, and responds to those fears with reassurances that scientific knowledge has found vaccines safe.

> Vaccine fears prevent children from getting immunized. Media stories giving attention to the dangers of vaccines, thimerosal issues, and the recall of the rotavirus vaccine raised parents' concerns about the safety of vaccines. No studies demonstrate an association between immunizations and autism, sudden infant death syndrome, multiple sclerosis, arthritis, diabetes, neurologic disabilities, deafness, cancer, or acquired immunodeficiency syndrome (AIDS). Parents question the need to vaccinate because the incidence of vaccine-preventable diseases is low. (Stanhope and Lancaster 2004, 631)

Skepticism about vaccines becomes a result of vaccines' own success and effectiveness.

In fact, a recent study of under-vaccinated children suggests that knowledge is not the key factor in vaccine non-compliance, which actually rests on attitudes, beliefs and behaviors (Gust, Strine, et al. 2004).

This supports the idea that acceptance of the narrative is potentially crucial for vaccination's successful implementation. Under-vaccinated children (those who have received some required vaccines, but not the complete course) are associated with poverty, mothers with low educational level, and racial or ethnic minority status. The factors that seem to be most important for children who do not comply at all with vaccination recommendations and requirements are very different: highly educated mothers, high income, and an acknowledged skepticism about vaccine safety. Though researchers have made much of this unvaccinated population (the group that intentionally rejects vaccines), it constitutes only 0.3 percent of the target population (Smith, Chu, and Barker 2004). Intentional non-compliance is very rare: very few people actively reject the narrative.

The health professions literature speaks with a harmonious voice about vaccines. The following is a small but representative sample of comments from the health professions literature. Hundreds if not thousands of comparable quotations could be culled from the medical and public health literature. Given a strong cultural narrative, one might expect some consistency, but the actual level of consistency over nine decades is truly remarkable. Professional medical and public health journals leave little room for doubt that vaccines are an amazing and unproblematic intervention:

> It is, however, *only* through the development of an HIV vaccine that we have any hope of ending the [AIDS] epidemic. (Berkeley 2001, emphasis in original)

> Next to clean water, no single intervention has had so profound an effect on reducing mortality from childhood diseases as had the widespread introduction of vaccines. (Howson, Howe, and Fineberg 1991, 1)

> The conquest of poliomyelitis had all the elements of an American success story: the focus on an objective so simple in concept and so obviously beneficial to mankind as to resemble the quest for the holy grail. . . . (Dowling 1977, 218)

> The best means for preventing [a rubella epidemic] is in the proper application of an effective vaccine. (Weibel, Stokes, and Buynak 1969, 226–29)

> I wish to state again that the best way apparent at the present time for controlling and stamping out diphtheria from our communities is to actively immunize all children under 18 months with toxin-antitoxin. (Zingher 1918, 494)

I am fully convinced from my past experience that the vaccine treatment of whooping cough is by far the best treatment that we have at our command for the disease, and that not only does it alleviate symptoms and cure the disease quickly but also in a measure prevents those complications of the disease that are apt to be so fatal. (Sill 1913, 442)

The earlier assertions of the value and importance of vaccines were part of an ongoing process of meaning construction—building the vaccine narrative—while the later examples embody and reinforce the narrative. The earliest claims dealt with in this book, about diphtheria vaccine, hearken back to still earlier narratives about vaccines against smallpox, anthrax (in livestock), and rabies. Those early vaccines remain important because they laid, if not a direct scientific basis, certainly a cultural foundation for the modern vaccination story.

Historical Background

In the 1720s, first in London and then Boston, small groups of physicians began trying to protect people against smallpox[5] epidemics by *inoculation*. This meant introducing a small amount of fluid from smallpox pustules into healthy people when an epidemic was expected. They based this radical practice on anecdotal testimony from Turkey that such practices reduced deaths during an epidemic. Inoculation had been used for hundreds of years in various places around the world (Parish 1965), but this marked its formal introduction into direct American medical antecedents. Some people died from these inoculations, and inoculated individuals could also become smallpox carriers, transmitting the disease to others. Nevertheless, the practice was judged a medical and economic success and became the first preventive medical intervention that mitigated epidemics (Melchert 1973). Inoculation also contained the seed of vaccination: a weakened (safer) dose of a disease that promised to protect against the full-blown disease.

Vaccines' eponymous history began in 1790s Britain, when Edward Jenner confirmed through an experimental test the country wisdom that exposure to cowpox (an innocuous disease and the source of the term vaccine—from *vacca*, Latin for cow) conferred immunity to the deadly smallpox. His discovery made him a hero of the medical profession, as well as a popular hero among some segments of the general population. His vaccine promised to protect against the deadly threat from an unseen, unpredictable, dangerous disease. Originally employed, like smallpox inoculation before it, as a response to epidemic situations, smallpox vaccine quickly came to be valued for its general protective qualities. Within twenty-five years of its discovery in 1796, mass vaccination programs had been implemented in Scandinavia, on the European continent, in North America, and as far as the Spanish Caribbean, with varying degrees of success (Schibuk 1986; Fenner 1989; Rigau-Pérez 1989; Nelson and Rogers 1992).

With essentially no treatments or preventives to offer patients for smallpox (or any other disease) through most of the nineteenth century, medical establishments eagerly embraced smallpox vaccination as a standard practice. Denmark, Sweden, and France each instituted a national program of smallpox vaccination, and quickly and easily gained almost complete coverage within each state (Schibuk 1986). In Britain a different situation applied. Adverse reactions to the vaccine (vaccinated children sometimes died), the use of an unpopular poor-law bureaucracy to enforce mandatory vaccination, and concerns about vaccination as a violation of religious beliefs combined with a general distrust of the medical profession (which had a reputation for attending death rather than for saving lives) to work against efforts to vaccinate the population. Anti-vaccination societies and political parties sprang up. Through the nineteenth century, Britain's mandatory smallpox vaccination policies weathered highly contentious controversies (Macleod 1967). By the late 1880s, when researchers began to propound a scientific rationale for its effectiveness (i.e., the germ theory of disease), smallpox vaccine had begun to pass from a revolutionary and controversial practice into a standard procedure. Epidemic smallpox had by then also begun to retreat as a threat (Porter and Porter 1988).

In the United States, smallpox vaccination experienced both widespread popular acceptance and violent opposition. The initial reaction was similar to the Scandinavian experience, but by the 1840s American acceptance and use of smallpox vaccine declined. A resurgence of smallpox epidemics during the 1870s sparked not only renewed efforts to vaccinate, but also sometimes-violent anti-vaccinationism (Kaufman 1967). Many opposed vaccination on principle, arguing that it violated the American ideas about individual liberty (freedom from government dictates) about personal matters. Aggressive practices by public health departments, sometimes colored by class-based or anti-immigrant prejudice, often generated strong anti-vaccination sentiments. In one example, Brooklyn public health officials used their powers to quarantine healthy people who refused to be vaccinated (Colgrove 2004). Groups like the Anti-Vaccination Society of America (one offshoot of British correlates) coordinated resistance to smallpox vaccination, and were instrumental

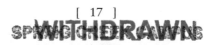

in some large-scale civil disturbances, like the month-long rioting that occurred in 1894 in Milwaukee, Wisconsin (Leavitt 2003).

The American federal system of laws meant that most compulsory vaccination laws were implemented at the state (or local) rather than national level. This made it possible for opponents to take on mandatory vaccination through incremental and local opposition. By the late 1870s, vaccine opponents had successfully repealed mandatory smallpox vaccination laws in states across the country. Another factor in the anti-vaccination movement's success was the considerable difference of opinion among American physicians about the safety and legitimacy of smallpox vaccination. This professional skepticism resulted in part from splits within the various branches of the pre-Flexner Report medical profession, but also because there were no established standards of proof for efficacy and safety. Through the 1890s, smallpox epidemics and anti-vaccination protests broke out in numerous American cities. As smallpox epidemics declined and public health agencies' authority to enforce vaccination policies gained legal provenance, smallpox vaccination changed; as smallpox became less virulent, vaccination campaigns (the main response to an impending epidemic) became increasingly less common, and therefore less intrusive in everyday life. The organized nineteenth-century anti-vaccination movement soon collapsed (Kaufman 1967).

Drastic reductions of smallpox epidemics and their reduced virulence, credited to smallpox vaccine, reified the value of the vaccine. The story of smallpox vaccine was based on an atypical disease, and one for which there was only sketchy systematic or objective evidence that vaccination by itself deserved credit for the end of the epidemics (Schibuk 1986; Hardy 1993). Nevertheless, the smallpox experience pioneered a path for development of subsequent vaccine preparations. By the late nineteenth century, the term vaccine became a catchword, certainly within the health professions community, for a safe and inexpensive preventive that averted dangerous epidemics.

Around the same time, evidence was beginning to mount that medicine was capable of doing more than presiding over deaths or taking heroic measures.[6] Pasteur's successes in the 1880s with anthrax and rabies vaccines, Koch's isolation of the tuberculosis bacillus, and the emerging germ theory of disease began to convert many of the remaining professional skeptics. The germ theory gave scientific and theoretical validation to what had previously been only an empirical claim: vaccination limited infection and saved lives. Public sentiment was important for these perceptions, and newspapers played an important role in creating public support for the regular physicians' enthusiasm for vaccination (Ziporyn 1988; Hansen 1998).

By the early twentieth century, vaccines and the nascent bacteriological laboratories that could produce them were beginning to gain in prestige and authority, just as new forms of scientism were beginning to overhaul the medical profession. The Flexner Report, commissioned by philanthropists and released at the beginning of the second decade, confirmed the shift of American medicine towards the German model that relied on university education and laboratory-based research; it also ensured the ascendance of allopathic physicians over homeopaths, Thomsonians, eclectics, and the rest. In fact, because vaccines were bacteriology's only preventive or therapeutic success at the time (Worboys 1992), the rise of bacteriological medicine could arguably be traced to the rise of vaccines. For the first time, smallpox vaccination had allowed American medicine to claim an effective preventive.[7] Vaccines also quickly became among the most fashionable enterprises in medical commerce. The prominence of vaccines in a 1912 advertisement by a corporate ancestor of Merck pharmaceuticals promised protection against diseases ranging from cancer to gonorrhea (Galambos and Sewell 1995). This suggests that vaccination had marketing appeal among both the general population and medical professionals.

Medical historians identify New York City's anti-diphtheria vaccination program at the beginning of the twentieth century as the point at which modern, scientific immunology began (Blake 1948; Rosenberg 1979). With the creation of bacteriological laboratories devoted to their development, vaccines became more than a simple success story. Vaccines became a powerful selling point in the development of these new institutions, and for this newest version of scientific medicine. This link between vaccines and Modern Science increased acceptance among medical professionals; vaccines provided a practical application of the germ theory and bacteriological knowledge in organized medicine's nascent pursuit of cultural legitimacy. The success of the anti-diphtheria vaccination campaign in New York from the early teens until the 1940s was in many ways more of an institutional and public success than a success by an effective anti-diphtheria vaccine. The period from around 1900 through the 1930s saw the establishment of the institutional bases for modern scientific medicine, including the reform of medical education (Berliner 1985), the solid establishment of public health departments and bacteriological laboratories (Maulitz 1979), as well as the final victories by allopathic, scientific medicine over other medical traditions (Rosen 1964; Starr 1982; Rosenberg 1992; Haller 1994). American medicine organized itself into a coherent, streamlined, self-governing profession securely based in epidemiological evidence, laboratory science, and the bacteriological model of disease (Tomes 2001). Following the

Second World War, antibiotics, which had earlier demonstrated their capacity to combat bacterial infections, became widely available. Penicillin captured the medical and public imaginations, much as the vaccine against diphtheria had done before the war. Within a few years, however, it became increasingly clear that penicillin and its cousins were ineffective against a newly discovered kind of microbe, the virus (Hughes 1977).

The dramatic success of polio vaccine in nationwide clinical trials and subsequent polio vaccination programs in the 1950s gave vaccines a public-relations boost that brought them back into prominence, both in the public consciousness and within the medical-scientific communities.[8] The anti-polio campaign was a success partly because it employed advanced fund-raising and publicity tactics, and because it resulted in a vaccine. Perhaps even more importantly, mass vaccination had shifted its aim away from immigrants and the poor back to another target population: American children. Children were innocent victims and polio vaccine (as well as subsequent vaccines against other children's diseases like measles, mumps, and rubella), promised to protect them. Though perhaps most famous for triumphs of vaccination, the 1950s were a time when the high prevalence of more deadly and socially devastating diseases, such as syphilis and gonorrhea, had been endemic for decades (Brandt 1985), alongside other recurring and growing health problems like tuberculosis, heart disease, and cancers.

After the Salk polio vaccine discovery and public success, the medical research establishment experienced a renewed flurry of vaccine development and enthusiasm, as had happened during the first decades of the twentieth century. This time, however, the profession was in its clear ascendancy. Anti-diphtheria researchers had scrounged for funding and worked to establish credibility and to justify the vaccine enterprise within an often skeptical professional community; polio vaccine researchers had relied on sponsorship from a major foundation to fight a frightening disease. By the late 1950s, however, researchers began to set their own priorities for the identification of diseases as vaccine candidates, rather than simply responding to epidemics or waves of public sentiment. Vaccine researchers set their sights on hepatitis, rubella, measles, and other common diseases. Their ability to mount mass vaccination programs continued to depend on epidemics, as with the rubella epidemic in the early 1960s, but with the expansion of federal research funding, the dynamics of the vaccine research enterprise shifted more decidedly into the hands of researchers (see Chapter 2).

In 1975 and 1976, the swine flu vaccination program resulted in a high-publicity vaccine failure. The U.S. Public Health Service developed and aggressively marketed an adult vaccine against swine flu, based on epidemiological predictions that an impending swine flu epidemic would be as devastating as the one that had swept through the population in 1918 and killed millions. The epidemic never developed. More importantly for the reputation for vaccination, the swine flu vaccine caused some highly publicized adverse effects that in turn highlighted technical difficulties that would otherwise never have become public. As a direct result, the Public Health Service's status within the federal administrative bureaucracy fell dramatically. Because critics framed the problems with the swine flu vaccine as a failure of policy, not science or medicine, the swine flu fiasco did not affect existing vaccination programs, and the policy missteps have not reflected badly on vaccines in scientific or medical terms (Neustadt and Feinberg 1983). Vaccines' status remained consistently high among physicians and the general public, and new vaccines continued to be pursued aggressively, if increasingly outside the structures of government.

In 1977, the World Health Organization and the Centers for Disease Control certified the eradication of smallpox; they credited it to the use of vaccines (GCCSE 1980; Henderson 1987). This supplied the long-anticipated conclusion to the narrative loop of vaccination: complete control of disease by eradication. Smallpox became the model for disease eradication programs, and raised expectations about the capacity of vaccination to remove rather than simply reduce threats of infectious disease (Schibuk 1986). Other diseases, from polio to rubella, were quickly slated for eradication on the smallpox model (e.g., Orenstein et al. 1984; Hinman et al. 1987). With the advent of the AIDS epidemic in the early 1980s, hopes for a preventive vaccine that would knock out the epidemic surfaced early and demonstrated considerable resiliency, despite discouraging results (see Chapter 4). Enthusiasm for vaccination continues, with the recent production of vaccines against chicken pox, Lyme disease, malaria, and other low- or no-mortality diseases.

Studying Vaccines

In the film *My Dinner With Andre* (Malle 1982), Andre Gregory presents a fanciful explanation to his dinner guest, Wallace Shawn, for why New Yorkers talk about leaving the city, but never do. New York City is a concentration-camp prison, he suggests, that the inmates (New Yorkers) cannot see because they are convinced it doesn't exist, even though they built it themselves. This is an apt model for conceptualizing dominant cultural narratives. The nature of any cultural narrative is that we are not generally aware of it, though it helps frame our worldview, and if asked about its plot or characters, we know them well. Empirical realities that do not fit the narrative's worldview appear dissonant and wrong. We can reject evidence before our eyes in favor of a confirmed expectation that conforms to the narrative. Narratives guide what we see and know. Sometimes, we see what is not there because of the expectations the narrative imposes—as in the personal accounts of civil rights participants that conformed more closely to the dominant narrative of social movements than to the facts of their experiences (Polletta 1998). For vaccines, we thoroughly accept the narrative (consider how comfortable and right the polio story feels). As a result, we tend to see what the narrative prescribes—and find it difficult to see or accept events or information that contradict it. Because of the narrative, we do not like the idea that there might be something different there, or that we are seeing incorrectly.

We can see around narratives if we try. The first step is to identify and describe the narrative. The cultural narrative of vaccines tells the story of a deadly disease that exerts a terrible toll in human suffering and death. Heroic researchers, working altruistically, marshal the forces of modern science to develop a simple intervention to ready the body's own defenses: a vaccine. Properly prepared, we can defend ourselves, just as our science demonstrates human mastery of death. Through the application of a simple, safe, and effective shot, we protect ourselves and set the disease on the road to oblivion. Our compliance with mass vaccination policies is a moral obligation that protects each one of us at the same time that we contribute to our common goal of eradicating disease. Our compliance is morally right, practically easy, and both scientifically and politically progressive. By explicit extension, those who oppose, refuse, or resist vaccination are ignorant, anti-science, and a threat to the public health. They, too, are part of the story—the "bad guys" who try to subvert our attempts to win the war, but whose plans are doomed to failure.

Perhaps this last part of the narrative helps explain why vaccines remain so under-studied and under-theorized, despite their widespread use and their prominent role in medicine, public health, and in the reduction in infectious disease. Epidemiologists, immunologists, and medical research scientists have studied vaccines as part of their quest to develop new, better, or safer vaccines, or as a way to increase vaccination compliance rates (e.g., Marcuse 1991; Santoli, Huet, et al. 2004). Scientific researchers have generally considered vaccines' meaning to be static over time, and concentrated on technical advancements and distinctions: viral or bacterial vaccines, live or killed vaccines, whole-cell or subunit vaccines. Their research is technical, and its positivist assumptions about science neither permit nor recognize alternative interpretations. Vaccines have been considered part of the forward march of science (e.g., Parish 1965), or, taking efficacy, success, and cultural legitimacy for granted, vaccines have been used for studying other social processes, like the diffusion of innovation (Hollingsworth, Hage, and Hanneman 1990). Popular controversies have attracted scholarly attention, both in historical context (Blake 1948; Schibuk 1986) and in more contemporary policy terms (Guthrie 1977; Silverstein 1981; Neustadt and Fineberg 1983). Through all the research on vaccines, the consistent thread remains that they are effective, safe, and necessary.

In fact, the dominance of the vaccine narrative makes it impossible to study vaccines from a social or cultural perspective without hearing demands from all parties to explain "where you stand." This is because there are two highly polarized camps that either actively support or oppose the narrative; together they constitute the lopsided vaccine debate. On the one hand, we have vaccine supporters. They include physicians, public health workers, the professional medical and public bureaucracies, and state and federal (and global) policy makers—a powerful constellation of institutions and authority (the general public is generally in this camp as well, though relatively passive about it). Their unanimity about vaccines as beneficent and necessary, coupled with almost no tolerance for dissent about vaccines' continued use, quickly marginalizes any opposition to vaccines. An honest analysis that questions the usefulness of vaccination—that does not make *a priori* assumptions about vaccines' positive value—risks finding itself lumped together with the most radical anti-vaccinationism.

That is not to say that researchers have always approved every vaccine or turned a blind eye towards negative laboratory or clinical evidence about vaccines, or that there is no dissent within the ranks of medical and public health professionals. But dissenters must be careful, lest they fall (or be pushed) into the anti-vaccinationist category, from which there appears to be little chance of escape or rehabilitation. In the 1960s, Graham Wilson, a well-respected mainstream British physician, wrote a carefully researched and rather dull book about vaccines and their adverse effects; he felt compelled to address precisely this issue by proclaiming that, "I want to make it abundantly clear that I am not an anti-vaccinationist" (Wilson 1967, 289). Part of this polarization stems from the continuing strength of the narrative, and the way it frames vaccines and vaccination as purely beneficent, and anyone who questions them as a crackpot.

On the other side, vaccine opponents seem equally dogmatic in their approach (vaccines are dangerous, overused and/or should be done away with), but tend to be more inclusive and more diverse. Eager for support for their beleaguered positions about vaccination, they adopt a catch-all approach to negative information about vaccines, and are prone to accept support from any quarter, often regardless of its cultural, scientific, or logical legitimacy. Another aspect of this end of the spectrum is that opponents will, for example, frequently cherry-pick information about vaccines for any negative comments or ideas, and then quote them for the greatest effect (usually out of context), often regardless of provenance or validity. This approach also discourages thoughtful, reasonable analysis about vaccines, for fear that the products of such work, however evenhanded, will become a tool in the hands of anti-vaccinationists. The overall result is a chilling effect on open discussion and research about vaccines; one must be for them or against them, whole hog.

This book strives to exist in the elusive middle ground, without taking "sides." Have vaccines been of enormous importance in the reduction of infectious disease? Clearly, yes. Do vaccines and vaccination policies deserve closer scrutiny, careful analysis, and perhaps modification? Again: clearly, yes. Just as clearly, recognition of the existence of a cultural narrative about vaccines means that we need to be able to question and investigate that narrative, without becoming its victim. A narrative's power to guide our thinking about vaccines means that it has an impact on how we raise our children, who should be allowed to attend school, what relationship exists between bodily integrity and public good, how we should spend increasingly scarce resources, and so forth. It would, indeed, be unfortunate if this attempt to view vaccines from outside the cultural heuristic either became co-opted by opponents of vaccination, or became marginalized as "anti-vaccinationist."

The persistent dearth of "external" research is particularly unfortunate, because at a fundamental level vaccines and vaccination are very interesting. For one thing, the preventive aspect of vaccines is at odds with the long history of traditions in American medicine. American medicine (and this is a thoroughly American account) is built around the allopathic model: curing with opposites, heroic measures, and individual treatment. At least in theory, every medical patient receives individualized care from a personal physician—doses calibrated and drugs or therapies adjusted to fit particular or even idiosyncratic responses and needs. Two different patients with the same complaint might receive different treatment from the same doctor, though, of course, health care does not always live up to this model (Szasz and Hollander 1956). Even quarantine is subject to interpretation and variability depending on the specific nature of the case (Colgrove 2004).

Vaccines work differently. A vaccine, particularly one used in a mass-vaccination campaign, is a mass-produced biologic that needs to be one-size-fits-all, or nearly so; the same vaccine typically needs to work across genders, races, ages, genetic backgrounds, and individual medical histories, not to mention different forms of the disease. Thus vaccines call for a higher (or certainly different) threshold of consensus about the efficacy and safety of any individual vaccine preparation. Of course, there are opportunities for some individualized application of vaccines, and there are vaccines designed for specific sub-populations. A fundamental difference remains: vaccination programs are designed only in part to protect the individual receiving the vaccine; unlike cancer therapy, surgery, or most antibiotic use, vaccines aim to protect the entire target population.

Regular (or allopathic) physicians treat fevers with antipyretics, pain with analgesics, and prescribe antibiotics to help kill germs that have entered the body. By contrast, the logic of vaccination means introducing a small dose of the *same* (or similar) thing that makes patients sick, much as homeopathic physicians do. Although regular physicians advocate a wide range of preventive measures in addition to vaccination (e.g. exercise, diet, vitamins), their main training and practice is in the treatment and cure of existing conditions; American cultural values, as well as historical trends, have made doctors the people we go to when we get sick or to stave off imminent illness. We do not generally make preventive visits to our doctors, though in some situations that has become less uncommon, most notably around natal care. Vaccines are an interesting exception: they aim to prevent disease (except in a therapeutic form, which has yet to yield much beyond hypothetical efficacy). They deal not with individual patients who have specific complaints, but with statistical rates of immunity in populations, in the hope of avoiding the need for treatment.

Public health, unlike regular medicine, has always been engaged with the attitude toward health that vaccination embodies. Research on public health, surprisingly, has relatively little to say about vaccines, perhaps because organized medicine has so effectively subsumed public health under its aegis (Fee 2000). Over the past four decades, sociologists, philosophers, and historians studying public health and medicine built new frameworks for understanding the social and cultural role of science and technology. Leaving behind the boosterism of hagiographic histories, and eschewing the distinction between "internal" and "external" realms in science generally (Shapin 1992), they have carved out an eclectic set of theoretical stances on research behavior and scientific development. They range from positivistic faith in the objectivity of the scientific method (Fleck 1979) through context-based analyses of science in dynamic interaction with society and culture (e.g. Longino 1990; Pickering 1992) to interpretations of meaning and history that interest themselves in analyses of constructed meanings (Latour and Woolgar 1986; Sawicki 1991). These perspectives have opened new possibilities for understanding the role of science, technology, and medicine in society. Still, vaccines remain largely unexamined.

This book applies the perspectives of the cultural study of science and medicine to vaccines. The task is to understand the origins of institutionalized beliefs, practices, and narratives, as well as how the narratives have in turn influenced cultural attitudes and structures. From this point of view, the extent to which vaccines have been responsible for the declines in mortality from infectious disease (a positivist approach) becomes less important. Instead of judging how we ended up with vaccination as opposed to some counterfactual history of disease control, and therefore focusing at an important level on the science of vaccination, this analysis looks at the arguments, evidence, and (with the addition of narratives) stories that convinced medical researchers that vaccines were the way to go. Far from abandoning empirical approaches to research on science and medicine, this analysis expands that approach to encompass cultural and discursive dimensions within a framework that values empirical evidence.

For people who believe vaccination is good, necessary, and fundamentally safe (most of us), an analysis such as this may look like criticism designed to undermine the scientific provenance of vaccines; it may appear anti-science, anti-progressive, and therefore dangerous. Asking questions about the cultural provenance of vaccines—even suggesting that there could be a cultural aspect to vaccines' provenance— pulls back a veil. It places vaccination under the same analytical microscope as more traditional objects of sociological inquiry like social class, capitalism, gender roles, medical institutions, racial categories, sexual behaviors, emotions, or any of the other areas upon which sociologists have trained a critical gaze. Putting vaccines under that microscope threatens our comfortable ideas about vaccines (just as sociological inquiry continues to threaten our comfort with established class, gender, and racial norms), but it does not threaten the public health. Looking beyond the everyday meanings and functions of vaccination for scientists enables us to understand how vaccines became dominant. That can help us re-evaluate our strategies for disease prevention and perhaps improve public health. The vaccine narrative characterizes attempts to change the way we view vaccination as an immoral attack on vaccines. A narrative that precludes its own investigation is an interesting proposition, one well worth exploring.

By any account, vaccines are important because they offer to reduce the risk of disease and death, and the discussion of risk runs through both the narrative and history of vaccines. The relatively new field of risk analysis has produced a novel perspective on vaccination. By asking about the nature and social construction of risk related to vaccines, risk analysts reject the assumption underlying so much discourse about vaccination: that it is an incontrovertible bargain and that to study vaccination critically is to undermine both vaccines and the public health. Of course, risk analysts also use vaccination as a case to explicate other concepts (Gabe 1995). But the risk perspective has allowed researchers to peek behind the "self-evident trans-cultural legitimacy" of the vaccine narrative, and recognize that some groups may have radically different evaluations than others of the nature of the risks associated with vaccination (Rogers and Pilgrim 1995, 85).

A cultural study of vaccines also serves as a means to understand some of the relationships between medicine and society: how cultural and social ideas influence and affect medical policies, and in turn, the extent to which medical understanding and policy have an impact on society. Vaccines inhabit many layers of the interaction between medicine and general society: they offer an ideal site for understanding and evaluating such issues as the social construction of scientific truths; the unacknowledged inscription of cultural and social (i.e. non-medical) values into medical policy; the nature of non-medical criticisms of medical knowledge; policies and issues of consent, objectivity, and fairness in medical research; and the rational value of medical and public health practices. Because international and global vaccination efforts so often follow the American model (and rely on American resources), the examination of vaccines within American culture helps inform our understanding of the global use of vaccination to combat disease. The last chronological case, involving HIV/AIDS vaccine research and policies, most directly illustrates some of the ramifications of the vaccine narrative beyond the American experience.

Vaccines may be conceived in a laboratory, in a stable (as with the first vaccine, smallpox), in the minds of policymakers, or in the hopes of sick people and their families. In all contexts, however, the amount of cultural work necessary to transform vaccines from an isolated idea, a brilliant breakthrough, or an arcane medical discovery into an active vaccination program—usually as part of a broad-based social policy— is of an entirely different order of magnitude than for other kinds of treatments or preventives. Given this, a master narrative for vaccines becomes both invaluable and quite possibly necessary to accomplish the goals of vaccination in the United States, particularly in a national culture that places such high value on individual autonomy.

Despite important differences in perspective, American medicine has warmly embraced vaccination and had to overcome some ideological and practical hurdles to do so. Effective mass vaccination demands a consensus within the professional community about efficacy and safety, as well as a mechanism to deliver vaccines to the target population. It also demands willingness among intended recipients of the vaccine to accept it. The nineteenth century history of smallpox vaccination in Britain shows what can happen when people reject vaccines. As Emily Martin argues, "accepting vaccination means accepting the state's power to impose a particular view about the body and its immune system" (Martin 1994, 194). It requires this and more: a willingness to subject oneself and one's children to the introduction of a foreign substance and any risks that entails for a community benefit. This is a much broader consensus than most other drugs or public-health interventions expect.

How does a sociologist collect data to study a seventy-five-year-old narrative that developed over decades? Ideas about vaccines began and have been sustained largely from within the health professions. Researchers, physicians, and public health officers read and presented their ideas in the professional peer review literature. Therefore, this book is based on data from that literature, which provides historicized ideas about vaccines written by the actors engaged in constructing and contending with meanings for vaccines. The telling accounts are the ones that were most influential (Crocker 1998) for readers at the time and, therefore, also for my purposes. Within the context of each of the four disease/vaccine cases, individual published items serve as informants. By relying on a qualitative content analysis of health professions literature, each of the four cases serves, in turn, as an informant about its historical period, and the nature and function of the vaccine narrative in that time.

Of course, the four vaccine cases are neither exhaustive nor comprehensive in detailing the full richness of the vaccine narrative or its history—but this is not a history of vaccination. It is an attempt to understand the origins, meanings, and impacts of the vaccine narrative in American culture. Researchers have attempted or developed hundreds of distinct vaccines against scores of diseases since Jenner's discovery in the 1790s, and each one holds the potential to be an interesting and important case study. Because all those cases are inherently idiosyncratic and come from particular historical periods, none is immediately generalizable: rubella cannot be a stand-in for measles, and HIV/AIDS vaccine research does not necessarily help us understand the specifics of malaria or hepatitis vaccination. Rather, the four case studies in this book connect the historical links of the vaccine narrative over time. They serve as important cases in their own right, but also as representatives of important phases of medical history, albeit imperfect representatives. The chance to conduct controlled case comparisons appears rarely in historical research (Tilly 1984), and vaccination is no exception. Together the four cases make a consistent argument for the formation, existence, and activity of a vaccine narrative using what John Stuart Mill called "agreement proof" (1884 [1843]).

Perhaps the most interesting (and difficult) aspect of studying vaccines is working with, through, and around the general belief that they constitute a cultural, historical, social, and moral good. This belief permeates both popular culture and the scholarly literature. This book asks us temporarily to suspend our ingrained sense of the rightness of the narrative that the polio example at the beginning of this introduction describes, in order to understand more objectively the role of vaccines in American life.

Through these cases, the book attempts to analyze something that all of us think we already understand. The affirmative cultural narrative about vaccines is so pervasive in American society that it is almost entirely invisible—and therefore unexamined. Widespread acceptance of mass vaccination has protected it from criticism (with interesting exceptions) and allowed it to flourish as a medical public health intervention unlike any other, sometimes despite viable alternatives. The strength of support for vaccines rests not—or not simply—on demonstrated results from vaccination campaigns, but also on a much more sociologically interesting concept: a cultural narrative (and one that has effectively deflected serious scrutiny). The narrative has also exerted its power over the medical and research community that helped author it and reaps benefits from it. How we as a society think and act about vaccines is the overarching outcome of the complex historical process of meaning construction. This book seeks to understand and explain the processes and ramifications of that vaccine master narrative.

1

Diphtheria Toxin-Antitoxin
The Birth of the Modern Narrative

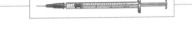

A Sanitary World

Perhaps the most feared disease of the nineteenth century was cholera. A gruesome disease that killed quickly, horribly, and randomly, without any seeming rationale, cholera was immortalized in Thomas Mann's *Death in Venice* as a way to show the depth of love for beauty and truth. For those of us lucky enough never to have seen a cholera epidemic, it is difficult to imagine the nature of the gesture that Aschenbach makes when he willingly stays in Venice to die of cholera. This brief description of the symptoms suggests how extreme such a sacrifice would be:

> *It is now possible to say with certainty that diphtheria can be prevented.*
>
> —Abraham Zingher

> Over 90% of cases are of the so-called *Cholera gravis* type. . . . The first stage, which lasts for three to twelve hours is of sudden onset with painless diarrhœa and vomiting . . . soon followed by agonizing cramps first in the limbs and then the abdomen. . . . [In] the second stage the signs of collapse increase. The surface of the body becomes colder and assumes a dusky blue or purple hue, the skin is dry and wrinkled . . . the pulse at the wrist is imperceptible. . . . In this condition, death often takes place in less than one day, but in epidemics . . . the collapse is [sometimes] so sudden and complete as to prove fatal in one or two hours. (Thomson 1969, 193)

Faced with a cholera epidemic, there was nothing to do but flee. But during the 1854 cholera epidemic in London, in one of the simplest and most elegant episodes of scientific inquiry, Dr. John Snow decided not to flee. Instead, he conducted a simple controlled study to test his idea that contaminated water was spreading the disease. By removing the handle from the Broad Street pump, he prevented people from accessing the water in that well, proved that cholera spread by contaminated water, and effectively ended the epidemic (Goldstein and Goldstein 1980). In this simple gesture, Snow not only demonstrated the value of empirical experiment, but the preventive power of sanitary medicine—the idea that clean air, clean water, and clean living could prevent disease. Cholera is no longer a public health problem in areas of the world where clean water is readily available.

At the time of Snow's cholera discovery, many of medicine's ideas still came from ancient texts. Aristotle's ideas, that sound health was the result of balanced humors, elements, and tendencies, survived the Middle Ages and persisted into the Industrial Revolution. That kind of holistic view of health persists, in forms, to this day. Of course we now know that germs cause disease, but most of us still believe that moderation and cleanliness are crucial to keeping disease at bay. People who believed in sanitary medicine—or hygienic medicine, as it was sometimes called—were able, like Snow, to effect sweeping improvements in public health without identifying the cause of disease beyond "filth" or unspecified products of still-mysterious processes. This meant that fresh air, clean water, and wholesome diet (variously defined) were of primary importance to good health.

By the late nineteenth century, a new recognition began to take hold that disease came from standing water (miasmas) or the fermentation process (zymotic disease). Behavior and environment were the most important factors, and the association between notions of cleanliness and health resulted in a hygienic revolution in health care. Rather than mystical or religious explanations for epidemics and seemingly random disease outbreaks, hygienic health theories reconstructed the causes of disease as the result of human filth, improper plumbing, and contaminated food and drink (Tomes 1998). In this view, health was a natural state that societies and individuals could maintain by simple adherence to good sanitary practices. As one sanitarian and an early advocate of a low-carbohydrate "fruitarian" diet put it, "Health is the undeviating expression of animal (indeed of all organic) life, always concomitant where the conditions natural to the animal are undisturbed" (Densmore 1892, 7). This kind of view of health and illness inspired public health programs that advocated better living conditions, indoor plumbing, and the clear separation of waste water (sewage) from drinking water.

Sanitary interventions were not, at least initially, conceived in small scale. The discovery that cholera could be transmitted to an entire community through its water supply made the transformation of water and waste systems imperative. This involved expensive and complex changes in the way large numbers of people lived, and substantial public investment. Moreover, the recognition that the environment was crucial to good health reached into all aspects of public and private life: housing-construction standards had to change and personal behaviors like bathing and cooking practices became subject to painstaking, expensive, and intrusive monitoring of people's everyday living. An outbreak of disease could trigger significant state action, in which quarantine and isolation measures often overruled individual preferences in the name of the public health.

For the first time, Western medicine had a guiding principle with a sound empirical basis as well as concrete recommendations for averting or alleviating the spread of disease. The belief in the importance of sanitary practices provided a set of guidelines upon which public health advocates could act, and those actions appeared to produce results. Rates of morbidity (sickness) and mortality (death) from diseases declined over the nineteenth century. Quarantine, which segregated the sick, slowed epidemics. The practice known as "stamping out" (isolation or hospitalization of patients, combined with disinfection) also proved to be of important use in mediating epidemics (Hardy 1993). By the end of the nineteenth century, it seems clear that most American physicians subscribed to the hygienic model of disease prevention—many held to these ideas well into the twentieth century. This was at least in part because sanitary medicine's general principles allowed for relatively easy adaptation to new information. When germs began to gain recognition for their involvement in disease, some sanitarians smoothly incorporated the idea, but did so in the context of a kind of behavioral quarantine: keep the germs away. Many sanitarians, however, rejected bacteriology altogether.

In addition to the general philosophy behind sanitary medicine and public health, other interventions were in common use and sometimes appeared to work. They ran the gamut from violent purgatives and radical surgery to small-dose homeopathic remedies and innovative treatments that involved, for example, the application of electricity to the body or massive quantities of water. Among these, one intervention gained special status—vaccination against smallpox.

Vaccines Work

By the 1890s, new developments in medicine and public health promised great things for the future, and Americans had already seen some important accomplishments. Vaccine successes—most notably smallpox—had made an enormous impact. Unlike other measures, smallpox vaccine prevented or reduced the severity of epidemics over the short term, and appeared to account for the general retreat of the disease. But the basis for that success—how smallpox vaccine worked—remained obscure. Explanations for vaccine effectiveness did not differ very much from explanations for any other remedies employed by doctors earlier in the 1800s, or in previous centuries. Well into the early twentieth century, cures and preventives (including vaccination) remained part of an established view of medicine as a holistic enterprise relating the body, health, and disease (Rosenberg 1979). Traditions of common use helped determine smallpox vaccine's weight and credibility, just as for purgatives, leeches, birthing practices, etc. A broad consensus agreed that mass vaccination against smallpox worked, but its success did not generalize to other vaccines. A narrative that encompassed vaccination in general did not develop until New York City's anti-diphtheria vaccination campaign of the second and third decade of the twentieth century.

Initial acceptance of mass vaccination had come quickly after Edward Jenner's discovery of smallpox vaccine in the 1790s. Based neither on laboratory tests nor on controlled epidemiological studies, acceptance rested on credible individual testimonies and broader subsequent experience that his cowpox vaccine conferred protection during smallpox epidemics. Advocates relied on a wide variety of means to persuade people to accept smallpox vaccination, ranging from admonitory rhymes to legislation, but they had no systematic or causal explanations for its apparent effectiveness; they had only stories of its success. Jenner described his vaccine this way:

> may I not with perfect confidence congratulate my country and society at large on their beholding, in the mild form of the cow-pox, an antidote that is capable of extirpating from the earth a disease which is every hour devouring its victims; a disease that has ever been considered as the severest scourge of the human race! (Jenner 1938[1800], 220)

For a century, the medical profession continued "beholding" smallpox vaccine's success without explaining its function. The notion that vaccines were an antidote, like Jenner's use of the word *virus* in his papers on smallpox vaccine to describe the thing that caused smallpox, was not technically meaningful. An antidote was simply something that stopped disease; no one had seen or confirmed the existence of anything called a virus; it was at that time just an idea. Like the evidence of efficacy, terms like antidote and virus conveyed little more than a descriptive sense of the vaccine's apparent effect. The most practical aspect of vaccines, however, seemed clear: they were effective at preventing death by smallpox.

Evidence of efficacy was entirely typical of the period: painstaking but not theoretically robust. Unable to explain why vaccination worked, Jenner focused on detailed description of cases when it did work, and instructions for how to introduce the "infectious matter" into recipients. Jenner's initial papers on smallpox vaccine recounted more than a score of detailed, individual successful uses of vaccine without explaining the mechanism by which the vaccine operated. In fact, throughout the nineteenth century, when vaccination established its initial reputation for preventing disease, no one knew what caused smallpox, how it was spread, what the vaccine did, or what the crucial ingredient in the vaccine was that prevented the disease.[1] Physicians and scientists did not develop a coherent explanation for smallpox vaccine's effectiveness until well after it had an established positive reputation. Only during the last third of the nineteenth century did researchers begin to hope for success using vaccines against diseases other than smallpox. This hope came with the development of the germ theory of disease.

The germ theory of disease revolutionized Western medicine, as laboratory researchers isolated and transferred germs—and as little of anything else as possible—and dissected innumerable guinea pigs for proof that disease resulted from specific, causative germs. The theory has become a commonplace: every disease is caused by a specific germ, the disease cannot exist without the germ and the germ has the ability—by itself—to cause the disease. The germ theory quickly began to contend with long-established disease paradigms, most notably sanitary medicine (though it also challenged ideas that disease arose from miasmas, generated spontaneously from filth, resulted from imbalances in the "humors," developed as the result of immoral behaviors, or had zymotic origins). Louis Pasteur's famous experiments in the 1860s disproved spontaneous generation, and his highly (but not unproblematically) public successes with rabies and anthrax vaccines brought widespread attention to him and his discoveries (Latour 1988; Hansen 1998). Further acceptance of the germ theory came in 1876 with Robert Koch's proof that a particular kind of bacteria was the sole cause of anthrax (King 1991), and his isolation of the germ that causes tuberculosis in 1882 (Fee and Hammonds 1995). Despite these laboratory breakthroughs, there were few applications of the germ theory through the end of the nineteenth century.

The outstanding exception was diphtheria antitoxin, which became available in 1895. Antitoxin was not a vaccine in the modern sense, though it did confer some immunity. A dose of antitoxin could cure diphtheria and confer a few weeks of passive immunity, immunity that depended on the continued presence of antitoxin for its strength. Unlike smallpox vaccine, which seemed to simulate the effects of surviving a case of smallpox, and appeared to confer lifelong immunity, diphtheria antitoxin's immunity was powerful, but short-lived. It was also the product of laboratory science—a practical application of the germ theory of disease. In fact, the diphtheria antitoxin program, spearheaded by the New York City Department of Health bacteriology laboratory towards the end of the nineteenth century, is the point at which medical historians mark the beginning of modern scientific immunology (Blake 1948; Starr 1982). For the first time, laboratories used the germ theory to produce an effective treatment. Antitoxin's stepchild, diphtheria toxin-antitoxin, became the first modern, laboratory-tested, bacteriological vaccine to be developed under the germ theory of disease and employed in a civilian population.

When the twentieth century opened, American medicine was poised on the threshold of modernity. As the new scientific methods of medical research displaced one theory after another, the germ theory promised (or threatened) to shift the ways professionals contended with disease. Not an abstract theory, the germ theory grew out of laboratory research and the reductionist view that reality could (and should) be broken down into its smallest parts in order to understand its essential qualities. Together with the new bacteriology labs, like the one in New York, the germ theory set the stage for radical changes in medicine and public health practices. Many sanitarians, who had long dominated public health departments and believed in the primacy of clean air, water, and healthful living conditions, initially rejected the germ theory (to their professional disadvantage) and increasingly found themselves marginalized as bacteriological methods came to the forefront.

In 1900, medical education institutions were as eclectic and unregulated as medical practice, and had no standard curriculum. Within two decades, however, reformers began to reorganize American health care to conform to the principles of laboratory science, and the regular (allopathic) physicians began to organize themselves into a powerful profession (Starr 1982). The Flexner Report, commissioned by John D. Rockefeller to map out the future of medical education in the United States, and promulgated and enacted during the second decade of the twentieth century, reorganized American medical education—and eventually practice—around the narrower, scientist-and-university-based system, of the kind used in Germany (Kohler 1979; Berliner 1985). This marked the beginning of the end of legitimacy for traditional (and varied) modes of thinking and practicing for health professionals. Despite these far-reaching changes in the underlying ideas and structures of American medicine, the germ theory had made little immediate impact on the practice of medicine or the prevention of infectious disease. That changed with the development of diphtheria antitoxin, a clear success that came directly out of modern laboratory science. Antitoxin, though highly publicized and widely hailed as a miracle cure, did not by itself directly change other aspects of the practice of American medicine.

A decade into the twentieth century, the same New York City Department of Health that had earlier led the antitoxin campaign, initiated an anti-diphtheria preventive vaccination campaign using diphtheria *toxin-antitoxin*. This brought together the new theoretical foundation for modern medicine (the germ theory), the single most effective intervention (vaccination), the new institutions of medical and public health research (bacteriology laboratories) and the modern public health department. The result was a diphtheria vaccine (diphtheria toxin-antitoxin) designed to wipe out diphtheria. Diphtheria toxin-antitoxin failed to achieve that goal, and Americans would have to wait until the early 1940s, and the acceptance and widespread use of diphtheria toxoid (a form of toxin neutralized with formalin, instead of with antitoxin), for a preventive vaccine that conferred immunity and prevented healthy carriers from transmitting diphtheria. New York's diphtheria toxin-antitoxin vaccination campaign did, however, transform the American vaccination narrative by bringing bacteriological science firmly and irrevocably into the vaccine story. Between 1910 and the mid-1930s the experience of and publicity about the toxin-antitoxin campaign became the template for the vaccination story we know today. That story was based in laboratories, the prevention of childhood disease, and an unimpeachable scientific provenance for vaccination.

Diphtheria Vaccine Writes Its Own Story

Diphtheria is a highly contagious respiratory infection that usually afflicts children. It is characterized by the development of a membrane across the windpipe at the back of the throat, a croupy cough, fever, nausea, and sometimes-serious complications caused by the diphtheria toxin that can affect the heart and the nervous system, and lead to death (Berkow 1997). This excerpt from an article published in the Journal of the American Medical Association in 1907 demonstrates the dangers associated with the disease, and exemplifies the established norm at that time for reporting research on diphtheria:

C.M., male, aged 13, developed diphtheria which was diagnosed as such April 11. On the afternoon of April 10, though the throat was most carefully examined, no membrane could be discovered. The following morning, however, it covered the tonsils, posterior pharynx, uvula and nasal cavity. The attack was apparently a most malignant one, cultures of pure growth of the Klebs-Loeffler bacillus being made from swabs of the nose and throat. On the night of April 12, the patient, while in a critical condition, was kissed by the three other children in the family and also by his parents; this in the face of severe opposition on the part of the attending physicians. The patient died April 13, having previously received 60,000 units of diphtheria antitoxin. (Purdy 1907, 2184)

The rest of the family received large doses of antitoxin (which had been ineffective for the boy), and survived. The article uses an individual case to ask questions about the kinds of antitoxin doses necessary to cure diphtheria. It brings the devastatingly quick nature of the disease into stark relief, and reports a "most malignant" case of diphtheria and the failure of antitoxin to cure it. The germ theory is in evidence, as the proof that this was a case of diphtheria was not in the symptoms, though they were typical and unique, but in the confirmed presence of the Klebs-Loeffler bacillus from a throat culture: the causative germ. If the antitoxin had worked—had cured the boy—this account would read rather like the accounts 110 years earlier that Edward Jenner compiled to make his case that smallpox vaccine was effective.

Two things in this excerpt are particularly important for understanding the nature and very existence of the subsequent toxin-antitoxin vaccination campaign. The first is the fact that eleven years after the introduction and widespread use of antitoxin, this family contracted diphtheria and one of them died from it. Antitoxin could (usually) cure diphtheria, but even its widespread use had failed to eradicate the disease, failed to avert scenes like the one described above. The second was the nature of the story presented. It conveyed some potentially clinically interesting information and ideas: a case in which antitoxin failed to cure diphtheria, the notion of stronger and weaker cases of diphtheria, and the fact that the physicians were unable to prevent family members from coming in close contact with the sick boy. But it remained an individual clinical case that spoke only about the specifics of the idiosyncratic case at hand.

The incomplete curative power and short-lived immunity provided by antitoxin spurred researchers to search for a longer-lasting preventive. This they believed they found in a carefully balanced combination of diphtheria toxin and antitoxin, called "toxin-antitoxin," which appeared to confer lasting immunity to diphtheria in guinea pigs[2] (Smith 1907). The prospect of life-long immunity to diphtheria galvanized public health officers in New York City, who determined to use a preventive toxin-antitoxin vaccine to solve the diphtheria problem: "we had a growing conviction that, wonderful as were the results of antitoxin, diphtheria could never be conquered by it" (Park 1922b). The search for a way to "conquer" diphtheria was the guiding force of the diphtheria vaccine campaign.

Researchers began the public campaign for mass vaccination by redefining diphtheria as a problem that needed measures beyond the widespread use of antitoxin. Part of that redefinition took the form of comparative rates, rather than tragic stories. As William H. Park, head of the New York City Department of Health Laboratory, saw it:

> There have been 120,000 cases of diphtheria treated in New York since 1893. At that time the mortality from diphtheria was 1.30 per 1000 population, while in 1912 it was 0.21. The morbidity from diphtheria in 1898 was 3.42, in 1903 it was 4.85; in 1904 it was 4.65; in 1912 it had fallen to 3.61. Thus it might be seen that with the use of antitoxin, the mortality rate has been greatly decreased but the morbidity curve has decreased little if any at all. This shows the need of some procedure that will lessen the incidence of diphtheria and the question arises as to whether active immunity will give enough benefit to be worth the trouble since active immunization confers immunity on about three-fourths or two-thirds of the children receiving the injections for a period of about a year. (Park 1913, 1214)

The contrast between this quotation and the one at the head of this section is stark: Park mentions no names, personal stories or even individual cases. Park's numerical take on the problem of diphtheria morbidity found a receptive audience. His question about whether active immunity will be "worth the trouble" was merely a set-up for the obvious conclusion (to his view) that a mass vaccination program was both necessary and would be effective. This article followed increasing attention in the health professions literature to the development of an effective preventive toxin-antitoxin vaccine (e.g., Heinemann 1909; Atkinson and Bazhaf 1909–10; McClintock and Ferry 1911; Brown 1912–13). Park's attention, however, was not limited to the immediate issues of diphtheria.

The anti-diphtheria vaccine campaign brought subtle but important changes in the purposes of vaccination. Where smallpox vaccine promised to prevent death during epidemics, and perhaps even stave off an epidemic, the new emphasis expanded the role of vaccination to shift the emphasis from mortality (death) to morbidity (sickness) as the measure of success:

> All seek some means of bringing about active immunity; for this would seem under present conditions of living to be the only means of controlling and limiting the spread of the disease. (Place 1913, 1215)

The argument that only a vaccine could control the spread of diphtheria changed the goal of preventive medicine. No longer was preventing epidemics and death the goal; now vaccination would become sufficient (and therefore necessary) for the conquest of a disease. Smallpox vaccination, though widely used, had not precluded established practices of quarantine and "stamping out." The goal in vaccine prevention of diphtheria was to stop anyone from getting sick, to achieve complete control of diphtheria, and to do it using only a vaccine. This implied a direct attempt to supplant the holistic sanitarian public health tradition.

In fact, the qualification of "under present conditions of living" in the quotation above signaled the change in priorities that the ascendancy of the germ theory facilitated: disease could now be attacked directly at the putative (and reductionist) source—the germ. As a preventive vaccine aimed at reducing morbidity, diphtheria toxin-antitoxin could make sanitarian public health efforts obsolete, to the benefit of bacteriologists and regular physicians. This is the direct ancestor of our contemporary belief that neither cold and wet weather nor improper clothing cause the common cold; those conditions do not matter unless the cold germ (which happens to be a virus) is present. Likewise, if diphtheria (and, by extension, other contagious, infectious, and potentially epidemic diseases) could be prevented by a vaccine, then stale air, lack of sunlight, poor diet, and the other evils addressed by sanitary medicine were rendered nugatory. The zeal to improve health by changing living conditions that dominated and motivated sanitary medicine met, in the germ theory and their bacteriological laboratories, a new force that seemed poised not only to prevent death and epidemics, but implicitly promised to end disease itself. Vaccines also promised greater professional recognition for physicians and came ready with both an empirical theory (the germ theory) and nascent but increasingly influential institutions behind it (bacteriology labs). Instead of protecting the public health in general by working through policy to improve sanitation, working conditions, and living conditions, toxin-antitoxin vaccination advocates proposed a new strategy: deal with the germs and leave the housing, water, and other concerns out of the medical equation.

Between 1908 and 1912, the New York City labs refined and began producing a toxin-antitoxin vaccine and increasingly argued in the professional literature for a mass vaccination campaign employing toxin-antitoxin vaccine. They presented diphtheria as a continuing problem that would find its solution in the laboratory and with a vaccine.[3] Initial results on diphtheria toxin-antitoxin proved encouraging: "If further use supports these early impressions then vaccine will probably find a definite place in the prophylactic treatment of diphtheria, as numerous indications for the use of such a means occur at once to the clinician" (Veeder 1914, 158–59). Technical concerns continued to be important —both for improving effectiveness and for reinforcing the individual nature of the vaccination. The logic of vaccination, though historically rooted in the prevention of epidemics, began to promise to protect vulnerable individuals despite—or perhaps more correctly, irrespective of —living conditions. This was important because coming down with a case of diphtheria was not just a health problem, it was also a marker of low social standing (Hammonds 1993). In place of correcting the social and environmental correlates of coming down with a case of diphtheria (which the sanitarians maintained had a causal connection), toxin-antitoxin vaccine promised to remove the risk of the disease along with the public stigma of contracting it. The discovery and acceptance of the Schick test (e.g., Stovall 1916; Zingher 1917) meant that researchers could promise to "detect the susceptible individuals, and control in a simple and yet accurate way the results of active immunization" (Park and Zingher 1915, 2217). With the Schick test it became possible to establish immunity and susceptibility to diphtheria in a generally healthy population, separate from an epidemic.

Medical and public health articles in health professions journals increasingly promoted germ theory responses to disease, but they did so with different standards of research. Perhaps the most important difference in the New York laboratory's articles on toxin-antitoxin was the heavy reliance on numerical (and sometimes, but rarely, statistical) treatment of the accounts of toxin-antitoxin use. The anti-diphtheria vaccination campaign revived the goal from the 1890s antitoxin effort: complete control (Maulitz 1979). The framing of this argument within professional health journals called for nothing less than that the forces of scientific research and bacteriology should defeat diphtheria in what worked, despite the reserved language of research, rather like a moral crusade.[4]

The new emphasis on the use of numerical and statistical evidence for testing remedies and preventives signified more than a simple methodological innovation. To these researchers, using numbers meant more rigorous science, and thus became part of the self-styled medical reformers' attempt to equate their numerical brand of science with high morality (Marks 1997). The anti-diphtheria vaccine campaign became an opportunity to crusade not just for complete control of the disease, but also for improvements in the way medicine worked in the United

States. The diphtheria vaccine campaign broke important new ground for the validation of vaccine effectiveness in the "scientific" nature of this new type of evidence. Edward Jenner had been exacting in his description and examination of the case studies that convinced him (and mainstream Western medicine) that vaccination could prevent smallpox; Jenner was, for his time, a consummate and meticulous scientist. Park and his collaborators used the emerging forms of scientific evidence and rhetoric to advance the use of diphtheria toxin-antitoxin vaccine, as well as the reputation of the New York laboratory and its staff. Reports about diphtheria vaccine rode (and to some extent drove) the scientific fashion that favored large-scale comparative experiments and laboratory findings over strictly clinical case-study reports. These kinds of perspectives on the problems of medicine were beginning to make their way into many aspects of medical practice, but the bacteriological labs found themselves particularly well situated to take advantage of the trend. Bacteriology laboratories would develop vaccines for use in mass vaccination campaigns that promised to achieve complete control—eradication—of disease.

Institutions and Rhetoric of Modern Vaccination

Beginning early in the second decade of the twentieth century, researchers began promoting a preventive diphtheria vaccine (toxin-antitoxin) and kept that agenda moving forward. This effort was led by Park, as director of the Board of Health bacteriology lab in New York City, which dominated the professional literature on diphtheria vaccination.[5] A crucial factor that accounts for their dominant presence was the existence of the New York City laboratory itself—it provided resources, access to a test population, and official standing (and a regular paycheck) for researchers (Blancher 1979; Hammonds 1993). Their high rate of publication in professional journals brought their ideas—and their names—to the national audience of researchers, public health officers, and regular physicians who read professional journals.

The toxin-antitoxin vaccine campaign began by introducing and normalizing the use of statistical information over a case-study approach. Park, his associate Abraham Zingher, and their assistants who worked at the New York City laboratory used the measured and cautious language of bacteriological science when they spoke to the professional audience. Park and his collaborators made no outrageous or emotional claims, and presented careful and precise documentation of their work.

Tables replaced personal description. Results and findings dealt with rates and proportions—"active immunization was noted in 25 to 30 per cent. of the injected individuals" (Park and Zingher 1915, 2217)—but refrained from mentioning individual stories, even when the number of cases was small enough to justify individual description, and too small to merit the discussion of rates. Gone were the detailed case histories that had convinced doctors of the efficacy of smallpox vaccine; there were no more sad (but personal) stories of individual cases, like the thirteen-year-old boy at the beginning of the previous section. Twenty-first-century readers need to do little interpretive work to understand what Zingher meant when he wrote, for example, that "85 per cent. of children from 2 to 3 years of age are susceptible" to diphtheria (Zingher 1922, 1945). But in the first decades of the century, this was an innovative way of writing about medicine and disease; it spoke the modern language of rates and stood in stark contrast to the clinical case-study approach. Its use in the context of diphtheria vaccine helped constitute the language of the health professions that we now recognize as typical.

The individual clinical report persisted in the literature, even after these more "sophisticated" kinds of evidence became more common in the journals, but they rarely generated follow-ups. For example, in 1924, a Connecticut physician reported an unusual reaction to a diphtheria toxin-antitoxin vaccination (and recognized the preeminence of the New York "authorities"):

> I am reporting this case because of the rarity of the condition. . . . None have come to my attention by report of the New York authorities who, in this country, were among the first to initiate this means of prevention and through whose hands an enormous amount of material has passed. . . . The rash was confined to the trunk and extremities. . . . the left arm from the elbow to the shoulder was slightly swollen, a deep uniform red on both surfaces. (Steele 1924, 1262)

Had the research on diphtheria toxin-antitoxin consisted of such reports, it seems unlikely that the mass vaccination plan would have come into being at all. By contrast, a typical article in the "new" mode, like this one by Park, recounts Emil von Behring's early discovery of diphtheria toxin-antitoxin, and the attempts to use it to immunize populations:

> The example of von Behring led Hahn and Summer shortly afterward to offer toxin-antitoxin to the 4,300 children [in] Magdeburg, where diphtheria was endemic. Of the 1,097 children injected, 633 received a full series of three injections; 255 received two injections, and 209 received one. . . . There was no difference in the development of cases of diphtheria among the treated and the untreated during the first

two weeks following the completion of the injections; but after that time there was a lessening of the number in the treated portion. (Park 1922b, 1585)

Here we have not the members of the family or community who survived, but the "treated portion" of the population.

Early clinical case studies could never provide the kind of population-based data that Park used to press the case for toxin-antitoxin as the solution to the diphtheria problem. An important factor in the ability of bacteriology to supplant clinical and case-study reports was the nature of the institution. In fact, only studies at a major, well-funded laboratory with access to a population amenable to testing of large-scale programs could produce such data. Though they used their laboratory to promote diphtheria toxin-antitoxin, Park and his colleagues achieved something much more enduring: the sense that the bacteriology laboratory was the place from which infectious disease would be defeated. At the same time, the necessary institutional context for bacteriology was easier to develop than sustaining many sanitarian traditions.

Unlike sanitarian public health measures, setting up a bacteriological laboratory was relatively inexpensive. Labs created the usual budgetary considerations involved in any kind of new appropriation, but a new bacteriology lab still cost much less than the wholesale changes in housing codes or infrastructure that sanitary medicine demanded. It also did not create the same kind of conflict with established interests in society. As the emerging class of physicians and bacteriological researchers left behind the social reform ethic that had been central to their professional climb to higher status, the laboratory was a natural destination (Feldberg 1995). The prospect of reducing the social problem of high morbidity rates from infectious disease without altering the fabric of society, while boosting their own prestige and professional status, made vaccines an even more attractive proposition to the physicians and researchers who were in a position to take advantage of it.

Increased funding for bacteriology helped the New York researchers accomplish their goals. As a result of political changes in New York City (e.g., incorporation of the "outer boroughs" in 1898) and changes in administration, the New York City laboratory dramatically expanded its range of operations and its budget. By 1910 the annual operating budget from the City alone was in the neighborhood of one million dollars, an unprecedented amount for that time (Imperato 1983). Over the succeeding decades, the fortunes of the laboratory fluctuated (Duffy 1974), but it maintained and even improved its reputation as a model among other health departments at all levels in the United States

(Imperato 1974). Later, the New York lab's leaders successfully solicited significant funds from non-governmental sources (Fee and Hammonds 1995). Acceptance and enthusiasm for the achievements of laboratory science migrated into the public consciousness only slowly. The diphtheria toxin-antitoxin vaccination campaign required a public-relations effort to enlist the support and cooperation of the people of New York. Though developed in the laboratory, vaccination campaigns had to be implemented in large populations.

The early use of numbers-based language came about in the context of vaccines and bacteriology labs for a reason. With diphtheria toxin-antitoxin, vaccines became a scientific, laboratory-based public health initiative, designed not for the individual patient (though, importantly, the benefits of immunity redounded to any vaccinated individual), but for the population as a whole. Vaccination was a medical intervention that was singularly accessible to epidemiological and statistical measures: its preferred use was in the mass, and therefore measures of effectiveness came easily in terms of rates. It mattered much less how any individual fared, because the goal was to protect the population, not just the individual. (In this, vaccination policies borrowed important concepts from sanitarian medicine.)

By itself, the existence of a bacteriology laboratory did not result in deep changes in preventive medicine. As the New York laboratory's researchers used the new kinds of evidence, they also aggressively advocated for the practical utility of active immunization by diphtheria toxin-antitoxin. In the progressive medical tradition that characterized scientific medicine and public health at the time, there was little equivocation about what needed to be done:

> Over 80 percent of deaths from diphtheria occur under five years of age. [In view of this] we have urged that every child from six months to two years of age should receive the active immunization with toxin-antitoxin. (Zingher 1920–21, 117)

and, again more clearly,

> Active immunization ... is essential in bringing up a diphtheria-immune population. ... Diphtheria outbreaks can be completely controlled in homes, institutions, and schools by promptly applying the Schick test and by giving prophylactic injections of antitoxin to the susceptible individuals. (Zingher 1920–21, 123)

These quotations leave the reader with little room for doubt that every child needs to receive the toxin-antitoxin, which is "essential" and can "completely control" the continuing problem of (still dangerous, though increasingly less lethal) diphtheria outbreaks. The language that researchers used varied, however, depending on the audience. Outside the realm of professional journals, they were still freer to make outsized claims about efficacy, and to indulge the enthusiasm they undoubtedly felt at the prospect of eradicating diphtheria.

In an article uncharacteristically unguarded for a medical journal, Abraham Zingher, writing for the New York laboratory, demonstrated the kinds of publicity techniques that New York was using for the fight against diphtheria. He quoted extensively from pamphlets distributed in New York City Schools to encourage parents to have their children vaccinated:

> *it is now possible to say with certainty that diphtheria can be prevented and that not many years hence there will probably be as little diphtheria then as there is smallpox now. . . . it is possible by means of three or more injections of a different* [than the Schick injection] *kind, given about a week apart, to "vaccinate" the child against diphtheria so that he will probably be protected against this disease for the rest of his life. . . .* One of the fine things about this method of diphtheria vaccination is that *children are not made sick by it,* as sometimes happens after smallpox vaccination and often after typhoid vaccination. (Zingher 1921, 338, emphasis in original)

In a subsequent article, Zingher reported the plans to go ahead with "an extensive diphtheria prevention campaign in New York City among children of preschool age." He described this plan as "an important preliminary step in any comprehensive campaign of diphtheria prevention" (Zingher 1922, 1952). The goal of the anti-diphtheria researcher/ activists remained to carry out their "comprehensive campaign" for the complete control of diphtheria.

Reports of the importance of toxin-antitoxin vaccination in the public press reproduced essentially the same information, but were less restrained in presentation. A *New York Times* article titled, "End of Diphtheria Assured by Experts," and with the subheading, "health department declares all children may be made immune," reported that by

> injection on three separate occasions at intervals of a week of a properly balanced mixture of diphtheria toxin and antitoxin we can produce without harm or danger a permanent immunity which will make the child invulnerable. . . . (NYT 1920)

Similar reports followed in the mainstream press, encouraging parents to participate in the anti-diphtheria vaccination campaign. The onus remained on the population to accept the wisdom of this purported miracle of science, which was consistently portrayed as entirely unproblematic and promising complete control. Newspapers through the 1920s reported the toxin-antitoxin advocates' idea that, "ignorance, superstition and prejudice still stand in the way of complete control of diphtheria" (NYT 1926). Emphasizing that diphtheria toxin-antitoxin held the promise of complete control and awaited only better coverage (better compliance) in the general population to accomplish that goal, reaffirmed the deviant (ignorant, superstitious, prejudiced) nature of non-compliance.

The Successful Failure of Diphtheria Toxin-Antitoxin

Researchers, newspapers, and public health officials from across the United States, and even internationally, hailed New York's toxin-antitoxin campaign as a triumph of science and progress against disease. The coordinated mass vaccination program used the Schick test to confirm immunity to diphtheria; that additional information made it possible to target diphtheria-vulnerable individuals and populations within the city. Unlike the experiences with smallpox mass vaccination in England (and, to a significant but lesser extent in the United States), which had led to rioting, created political unrest, and contributed to long-standing mistrust of medical authorities, the toxin-antitoxin campaign had been characterized by peaceful, careful, and supportive compliance. Diphtheria toxin-antitoxin worked—in laboratory tests, in field use, and among the general population. Just as the Schick test could verify an individual's susceptibility to diphtheria, the mortality and morbidity rates for diphtheria verified that toxin-antitoxin vaccination had begun to signal the end of diphtheria in New York—and by extension, the United States and the world. It was a triumph for the germ theory, for laboratory science, and for the individual researchers who had dedicated decades of their careers to the "complete control" of diphtheria.

By the early 1930s, however, after the mass vaccination of hundreds of thousands of New York City schoolchildren and a steady decline in both morbidity and mortality, diphtheria death rates began once again to increase (NYT 1932). Researchers began to recognize that although credited with some reduction in diphtheria morbidity, toxin-antitoxin was no more capable of eradicating diphtheria than antitoxin had been (Duffy 1974, 560; Hammonds 1993, 254–56; Fee and Hammonds 1995). This led to one of the more important technical discoveries that came out of the toxin-antitoxin vaccination campaign, the clarification of the problem of healthy carriers—that people who were not sick themselves continued to spread the disease despite being immune themselves (Ziporyn 1988). Researchers had failed to anticipate the fact that neither antitoxin nor toxin-antitoxin had any effect on diphtheria carriers. This indirectly reinforced the fact that vaccines rarely protected all individuals: their strength was in creating herd immunity. The idea that humans could and would completely control diphtheria persisted, and in the late 1930s Americans began to make the switch from toxin-antitoxin to diphtheria toxoid (a form of toxin weakened with formalin, rather than with antitoxin), which had been developed a dozen years earlier and been in widespread use in Canada since 1926. Only with the widespread introduction of diphtheria toxoid in the United States was the diphtheria-carrier problem overcome. Diphtheria toxoid remains part of the trivalent diphtheria-pertussis-tetanus vaccine currently in wide use, and in that form, a diphtheria vaccine remains a fixture in the public health requirements throughout the United States.

The outcome of the toxin-antitoxin vaccination campaign itself, however, was not complete control. In fact, despite the highly touted importance of "bringing up a diphtheria-immune population," it is not clear that there were all that many children who needed to be vaccinated in order to be safe from diphtheria. Researchers admitted publicly (but discreetly) quite early that the careful application of the Schick test for susceptibility to diphtheria revealed that about two-thirds of children were already naturally immune to diphtheria (NYT 1920). What the toxin-antitoxin vaccination campaign did accomplish was to institutionalize and instantiate the practical application of mass vaccination as the best way to prevent contagious diseases. The diphtheria toxin-antitoxin campaign established a new story for how vaccines "worked" and how to use them; after the toxin-antitoxin campaign, mass vaccination became central to the control of infectious disease. It established the precedent for the mass vaccination of whole populations absent high mortality rates or the imminent threat of epidemic, and inaugurated bacteriology, laboratories, and the new forms of evidence as central and essential ingredients of preventive medicine and public health.

Although toxin-antitoxin vaccine failed to eradicate diphtheria, the commonsense interpretation of the historical events remains that the bacteriologists were fundamentally right. Indeed, the New York laboratory earned its fame as a model for subsequent public health efforts: diphtheria vaccine had shown evidence of efficacy in large-scale tests, the disease was still a health problem, and even if researchers' claims about eradication and life-long immunity were overblown, they neither falsified nor exaggerated their data. The fact that pursuing a vaccine fostered professional interests weakened neither the effectiveness of the toxin-antitoxin vaccine nor the validity of the objectives that led researchers to pursue its widespread use. These were honest researchers dedicating their careers to preventing disease in a world in which—as in so many nineteenth-century novels—a cough early on could foretell death from an infectious disease by the end of the story. In fact, the early history of diphtheria vaccine seems by itself to substantiate the continued use of vaccination, and seems more a validation of the narrative of vaccines than anything else. It appears that the New York laboratory laid a solid foundation for establishing new policies and practices for the elimination of infectious disease by mass vaccination.

Told on its own, we can feel the resonance of the diphtheria toxin-antitoxin vaccine story—it fits as the early case of a vaccine that worked well, though not quite well enough. A brief comparative look at pertussis vaccine—in many ways a comparable disease vaccine case, but with a different short-term outcome—raises questions about what, precisely, succeeded in the toxin-antitoxin campaign. Why, since toxin-antitoxin lacked the ability to prevent healthy carriers from transmitting the disease, was it so widely used and regarded as successful? A comparative case highlights the factors that made diphtheria toxin-antitoxin, rather than any of the other vaccination efforts that were underway around the same time, so important for our culture's view of vaccines. The comparison reinforces the idea that the success of the toxin-antitoxin campaign may have hinged on institutional and discursive clout, rather than a revolutionary preventive that paved a new and successful technique for contending with infectious disease.

The Pertussis Vaccine

Pertussis (also called whooping cough) is, like diphtheria, an extremely contagious respiratory disease. Also like diphtheria, pertussis afflicts primarily children, but causes its highest mortality among children younger than twelve months of age. Another important difference is that pertussis transmission was harder to control using existing sanitary methods like quarantine: unlike diphtheria, pertussis is difficult to differentiate from numerous other conditions during the early—and most infectious—period. Only after the appearance of the characteristic "whoop" (created by the quick gasping intake of air after a prolonged bout of coughing), usually in the third or fourth week of the disease, was positive identification possible—and this was well past the infectious period. The early history of the preventive vaccines for pertussis is also similar.

In 1906, when diphtheria mortality was already largely under control through widespread use of antitoxin, two French bacteriologists isolated the germ believed to cause pertussis and developed a vaccine serum to treat and prevent the illness. By 1912, pertussis vaccine preparations were widely available from commercial sources (Galambos and Sewell 1995). As early as 1910, American health professionals began to show serious interest in preventing pertussis. One reason for this was that the relative number of whooping cough deaths had begun to exceed those "from diphtheria since the general use of antitoxin" as a treatment (Levy [in Grandy 1909]). Through the late teens, researchers and physicians continued to explore ways to contend with pertussis, but failed to reach a consensus about the best methods. Strategies ranged from aggressive pro-vaccinationism, to agnostic appeals for a case-study approach. The unifying professional consensus was that pertussis posed a grave threat to the public health (e.g., MacEvitt 1910; Sill 1913a, 384; Sill 1913b; Huenekens 1917, 1918; Luttinger 1917; Von Sholly, Blum, and Smith 1917; Bogert 1918; Barenberg 1918).

There was no clear consensus about pertussis vaccine, however. Some researchers were initially tentative in their embrace of a preventive pertussis vaccine, seeking more evidence about efficacy (Wollstein 1909). Some researchers advocated pertussis vaccination solely based on the dangers of the disease, which was "unquestionably so great that no therapeutic measure should be disregarded until after a thorough trial it proves of little or no value" (Hartshorn and Moeller 1914, 586). One researcher found his results inconclusive, but closed his discussion, in good empirical tradition, with the idea that "the treatment is worthy of further trial" (Ladd 1912, 584). Others felt more strongly, and wanted to move forward quickly with testing: "The results obtained in these twenty-four cases warrant, in my opinion, a more extensive trial of the [pertussis] vaccine" (Graham 1911, 166). Prior to the normalization of large-scale tests to demonstrate efficacy for diphtheria toxin-antitoxin, success in a trial of twenty-four patients might have been substantial evidence that pertussis vaccine was effective enough to begin general use. Given the evolving nature of acceptable proofs, however, support in the literature for pertussis vaccine built slowly over the succeeding decade, partly because there was no large-scale effort to test pertussis vaccine in a population.

By the middle of the second decade of the twentieth century, just as diphtheria toxin-antitoxin was gaining significant attention in the professional discourse, clinical and anecdotal evidence built up that pertussis vaccine worked—it could prevent the disease. Further case studies included strong claims for its usefulness (Hess 1914) and an increased certainty that pertussis vaccine showed promise, as this physician indicated in 1916:

> If the vaccines prove to have the value in prophylaxis and in treatment which the results of the last two years suggest that they may have, the control of whooping cough will be a simple matter. (Morse 1916, 727)

Numerous such reports came from individual public health officers or practicing physicians, though they presented clinical—not laboratory or epidemiological—evidence. The American Medical Association's Council on Pharmacy and Chemistry agreed that pertussis vaccine showed important promise, and in 1914 added it to their list of tentative remedies (Felton and Willard 1944).

Between the 1914 AMA approval and 1920 there was intensive interest in a pertussis vaccine, and by 1917, pertussis vaccine seemed to be following closely in the tracks of diphtheria toxin-antitoxin, with thirty-eight English-language articles relating to pertussis vaccine reaching publication. Many articles reported strong successes with vaccine (Grandy 1909; MacEvitt 1910; Sill 1913a,1913b; Hartshorn and Moeller 1914; Hess 1914; Morse 1916). A Rochester, New York health officer reported success in a pertussis vaccination campaign in that small city:

> [W]e do believe that through preventive inoculation for whooping cough, as carried on here and elsewhere, the disease may be materially diminished in virulence and limited in the number of children which it attacks.

The author credits this success to

> a booklet on whooping cough, advertised in the street cars in English, Italian, and German, and distributed the vaccine to physicians without cost. . . . Such is the beginning of a new era of preventive medicine, which is taking hold of the people; and one of these days we are going to vaccinate children against every disease "what they can be vaccinated against. "[6] (Goler 1917, 411–12)

Others used less informal language to make their case for pertussis vaccine (Huenekens 1917, 1918; Luttinger 1917). One group of researchers reported that, based on their controlled study, "we can be sure that pertussis vaccine conferred immunity" (Von Sholly, Blum, and Smith 1917, 1455–56). Still others reported successful and positive clinical experiences with pertussis vaccine (Bogert 1918; Barenberg 1918).

Despite, however, their promising results and the rising importance of pertussis as a disease, these reports failed to generate widespread support for a mass vaccination campaign to apply and certify the vaccine's effectiveness, and interest in pertussis vaccine did not sustain itself. From 1921 to 1927, there were only thirteen English-language articles on the topic of pertussis vaccine. The vaccine became one of a variety of alternative preventives and therapies that emerged as part of the scramble for an effective preventive or treatment; pertussis remained a dangerous and deadly disease. More than a dozen articles evaluated and advocated for diverse methods for contending with the disease including "the X-Ray," intramuscular injections of ether, and high-altitude airplane flights. Beginning in 1919, articles began reporting evidence about pertussis vaccine as a treatment (rather like diphtheria antitoxin) rather than a preventive (Bloom 1919; Reynolds 1919). This was doubtless related to advocacy for "therapeutic vaccines" by prominent public health officers like the Massachusetts Board of Health's star, Dr. Almoth Wright (comparable in stature to New York's Park). Wright believed that vaccines could be used to induce protective and curative immunity in people already sick.[7]

Some supporters of pertussis vaccination used the same kind of scientific rhetoric as Park had used to advocate for its widespread use. Thorvald Madsen, an Australian researcher-physician, made a brief splash in the professional literature when he articulated the problem posed by pertussis using the same style of presentation that had been so successful for the New York labs. He portrayed the problem of pertussis morbidity as one of rates that were too high:

> In the years from 1875–80, almost 85,000 died of whooping cough in Prussia alone; in England and Wales, from 1858–65 more than 120,000. The annual death rate in the United States registration area from whooping cough for the years 1912 to 1921, inclusive, was 10.25 per 100,000 population. When to these figures we add the fact that whooping cough may be accompanied by serious pulmonary complications, and that it may arouse a latent tuberculosis, we may perhaps realize how large a number of catastrophes may be credited to the account of this disease. There is, then, every possible reason to control whooping cough. (Madsen 1925, 53)

Like Park before him, Madsen also had a clear idea of how to control whooping cough. Later in the same article, he argued that pertussis vaccine presented "a remedy which takes the sting out of whooping cough" (Madsen 1925, 60).

But expressing the need for and efficacy of pertussis in the language of rates and populations alone was not enough to prosecute a mass vaccination campaign. Despite the consensus about the need for and the apparent effectiveness of early pertussis vaccine preparations, and after an extraordinarily lengthy trial period, the same AMA Council that earlier had accepted pertussis vaccine, recommended in 1931 that pertussis vaccine "be entirely omitted from New and Nonofficial Remedies" (Felton and Willard 1944). Only at the end of the 1930s, when bacteriology laboratories took up the cause, did pertussis vaccine achieve widespread acceptance among health professionals.

The rebirth of interest in pertussis vaccine can be traced to the involvement of institutionalized centers for bacteriological research that were capable of dedicating the substantial resources necessary to conduct "a large series of cases properly controlled and followed for a sufficient period of time" (Shorr 1936, 53). Beginning with a series of bacteriology-based publications by a suburban Chicago physician-researcher (Sauer 1933a, 1933b, 1935, 1937), the mid-1930s ushered in a renaissance of interest in pertussis vaccine. Under the reform-minded and pro-science Roosevelt administration in Washington, various cities across the United States began to imitate the model set by the New York City laboratory, as federal money flowed to fund research laboratories around the United States (Rosen 1965). The advancement of pertussis vaccine in the literature and in actual use depended on this proliferation of bacteriology labs and public health departments.

Though other labs contributed to the research that established the bacteriological foundation for the use of pertussis vaccine, the Michigan Department of Health stands out for prioritizing pertussis vaccine and adopting it, much as the New York laboratory had adopted diphtheria vaccine (Kendrick and Elderling 1935, 1936, 1939; Kendrick 1975). Together with supporting reports from bacteriology labs sprouting up across the United States, researchers achieved for pertussis vaccine what the New York laboratories alone had done for diphtheria vaccine. By the mid-1940s, just about the same time that diphtheria toxoid vaccine supplanted toxin-antitoxin vaccine, pertussis vaccine joined diphtheria as part of the recommended vaccination schedule for all American children. The AMA's Council on Pharmacy and Chemistry seal of approval certified the preventive pertussis vaccine and its place in the standard armamentarium of modern bacteriological public health (Felton and Willard 1944).

The comparison between the diphtheria and pertussis cases, though imperfect, reveals the centrality of laboratory sponsorship for the success of particular vaccination campaigns—both in the professional literature and in terms of vaccine use. The popular and highly regarded toxin-antitoxin vaccine became the model for subsequent vaccination campaigns against infectious disease despite its failure to achieve its goal of complete disease prevention. The apparently efficacious pertussis vaccines (more than one vaccine preparation existed during the early period), however, languished for decades. The discursive and institutional support that became available in the late 1930s allowed pertussis vaccination to achieve widespread acceptance within the health professions community.

Evaluating the Origins of the Modern Vaccine

Diphtheria and pertussis, two similar respiratory childhood diseases, had roughly comparable vaccines available and each generated similar levels of concern among health professionals, to judge by the professional literature. Both diseases seemed a natural fit for a preventive vaccine—pertussis even more so than diphtheria, because of the inherent difficulties in diagnosing pertussis and the existence of an effective treatment for diphtheria (antitoxin). The important difference between the two vaccine/disease cases appears to have been the strong institutional support for research and promotion of diphtheria vaccine—and its absence for pertussis vaccine. The ability to dominate the professional literature with large studies enabled researchers who believed that toxin-antitoxin vaccination was the way to achieve complete control of diphtheria to propagate a story that concluded with the "End of Diphtheria," as newspapers reported it (NYT 1920).

The idea that a weakened or smaller dose of an illness can confer immunity to that illness has been around for centuries, sometimes called variolation, inoculation, or other names. Jenner's discovery of smallpox vaccine in the 1790s formalized it in a way that health professionals could accept and use to avert or ameliorate epidemics. Other vaccines—against anthrax (in animals), rabies (as a treatment), and in the military (typhoid)—had been developed and used, but aside from the general idea of preventing disease, each failed to rise to the level of a paradigmatic model for subsequent vaccine efforts. The toxin-antitoxin vaccination campaign in New York was different. The efforts and experiences of the New York laboratory became the model for developing and implementing a mass vaccination campaign (Duffy 1990). The sequence was clear: employ laboratory techniques to identify the germ, develop a viable vaccine, test it in the general population, establish policies for mass vaccination, and begin eradication of the disease. This became the story of vaccines from that time forward: a story of logical and progressive research, science, discovery, and success. The comparison to the early course of pertussis vaccine illustrates some of the factors present in the toxin-antitoxin case that made it different—factors outside the accepted narrative, but factors essential to the narrative's success.

As one public health officer from Chicago outlined the situation before the toxin-antitoxin campaign had begun, the most important concern was "[h]ow to keep alive the aroused public sentiment towards ... diphtheria as it did towards smallpox" (Rawlings 1910). This is precisely what the researchers at the New York labs accomplished. "[Physicians] must utilize another practical method of immunizing against diphtheria. ... we may finally be able to get control of the disease that continues to be one of the biggest issues of preventive medicine" (Finnegan 1920). Diphtheria's "bigness" made it an important site for diphtheria vaccine advocates—at the same time that the same advocates worked to make diphtheria "big." Health professionals constructed the meaning of diphtheria as a threat to the public health based on new criteria (morbidity, rather than mortality) and they constructed its cure and preventive as part of their understanding of bacteriology. They also re-aligned the role of public health measures in controlling disease, by supporting vaccines in general, as well as the criteria by which all of them should be evaluated. Unlike pertussis vaccine, which lacked the kind of resources and institutional attention the New York labs brought to bear, diphtheria vaccination achieved national and international attention. That attention also translated into a foundational story of success.

The contrasting outcomes of the initial pertussis and diphtheria vaccine efforts suggests that their different early stories resulted from more than differences in simple efficacy. The interpretation of evidence about efficacy depended on the changing standards of proof, the status of the researchers producing the evidence, and the existence of an institutional sponsor for the vaccine. These factors also served to reinforce one another. In a sense, the development of bacteriological laboratories acted like an intervening variable between the diseases and the professional responses. Strong institutional support from the New York City laboratory for the "bacteriological option" (vaccination) made a vaccine the prevailing solution to the diphtheria problem, even though the featured vaccine candidate proved to be unsuccessful in an important way. When comparable kinds of institutional support for pertussis vaccine came into being by the 1940s, it also achieved the same kind of standing among health professionals and took its place among American medical and public health success stories. That is the lasting legacy of the early vaccination efforts to eradicate diphtheria. The most important outcome of the toxin-antitoxin vaccination campaign was not the vaccine preparation that researchers used in the campaign—it was the *story* that made the campaign into the kind of success that could be touted as "second only to clean water" in importance.

2

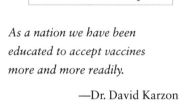

Rubella (German Measl~
The "Cultural Provenance" of Vaccination

■An Epidemic
of Birth Defects

As a nation we have been educated to accept vaccines more and more readily.

—Dr. David Karzon

Beginning in the spring of 1964 and continuing into 1965, the United States experienced its largest recorded rubella epidemic.[1] First on the east coast, and then several months later in the far west and Hawaii, American doctors began reporting high numbers of children born deaf or with vision problems. It soon became apparent that the United States was in the grip of a nation-wide epidemic—of birth defects. Scientists quickly concluded that rubella was the cause. At the time, estimates of the number of people affected ranged as high as 50,000 (Schmeck 1965), though epidemiologists soon reduced that to the consensus figure: 20,000 children were born with some kind of birth defect traceable to their mothers having been exposed to rubella during pregnancy (Neff and Carver 1970). The most common birth defect was deafness, followed by cataracts that could cause blindness (Gruenberg, Lewis, and Goldston 1986).

Rubella, popularly known as German measles, had for more than a century been recognized by doctors as a distinct disease, and there had been smaller, more localized, outbreaks. Until the 1964–65 epidemic, however, the disease had received almost no public attention. Unlike smallpox, rabies, diphtheria, or polio, which often kill, rubella's symptoms are mild, non-specific, and often entirely sub-clinical: a reddish rash and a mild fever. Rubella is difficult to diagnose, but harmless to the person who has it: no one dies of rubella (Wesselhoff 1947; Parkman, Buescher, and Artenstein 1962; Spock 1971). During a local outbreak in 1963, the director of New York City's Bureau

Preventable Diseases described rubella as "normally innocuous," though he acknowledged, "it could cause birth defects in children whose mothers came down with it in the first three months of pregnancy" (Schanberg 1964).

It was rubella's ability to cause birth defects that made the disease an important medical, public health, and social problem—and an unconventional vaccine case—without which the large rubella epidemic would have been little more than a nuisance and would likely have passed without notice and certainly without any organized response. In fact, rubella's symptoms are so mild that a rubella diagnosis can easily be uncertain and it is very possible to miss the symptoms entirely. Documented reports of rubella exist from as early as 1815, but it was not identified as a distinct and separate disease until over fifty years later (Manton 1815; Veale 1866; Emminghaus 1870). For seventy years after that, rubella was a disease entirely unimportant to any medical establishment—except to the extent that misdiagnosis would sometimes confuse it with the more dangerous measles or scarlet fever. In 1941, however, an Australian ophthalmologist noticed a correlation that looked like a causal connection between rubella in women during early pregnancy and congenital cataracts in the children born to those women (Gregg 1941). Subsequent research seemed to confirm the causal hypothesis about rubella and congenital defects (Swan et al. 1943), and the constellation of birth defects associated with rubella in women during the first trimester of pregnancy was named Congenital Rubella Syndrome (CRS). Except for the fact that rubella can cause birth defects, it holds little interest for medical practitioners and researchers. As one rubella vaccine researcher put it, rubella "was disparaged until 1941 when it received the imprimatur of greatness" (Forbes 1969).

In the mid-1960s, the fact that thousands of children had been born with birth defects galvanized the federal government and health institutions to act quickly and decisively. The epidemic became the precipitating event in the quest for a rubella vaccine, much as the big polio epidemic in 1952 had been for a polio vaccine. The parallels between the epidemics seemed obvious. A *New York Times* article conveyed the consensus among researchers, policy makers, and the general public that "rubella's ravages can only be ended when a vaccine makes German measles as scarce as polio has become in recent years" (NYT 1965b). Epidemiologists reported that rubella epidemics occurred in six-year cycles, with an especially large epidemic to be anticipated approximately every two decades: the United States should expect another, probably smaller, epidemic to begin in 1970 (Witte et al. 1969). This set a clear and short deadline for the development and deployment of a rubella vaccine. There was no dissent in medical or public health circles from the conclusion that the "best means for preventing [the effects of the anticipated 1970–71 rubella epidemic] is the proper application of an effective vaccine" (Weibel et al. 1969, 226). The polio and rubella epidemics had each set in motion stories that everyone hoped would end the same way: setting the diseases on the road to eradication.

Following a crash campaign to find a vaccine on such a short time-table, doses were distributed and administered across the United States. When the feared 1970–71 epidemic did not develop, researchers quickly hailed the program that the epidemic had set in motion to develop and deploy effective rubella vaccines as a success (PHSACIP 1971). Physician and public health organizations in the United States have since consistently recommended rubella vaccination for all children (Kunz 1982; AAP 1994), and rubella vaccine has been incorporated into the trivalent measles, mumps, and rubella (MMR) vaccine, with compliance typically monitored at the point of entry into public schools: no proof of vaccination, no school. Rubella vaccination has also become part of global public health initiatives against birth defects, such as the World Health Organization's "Expanded Programme on Immunization" to vaccinate children in developing areas of the world (EPI 1991). There have been no rubella epidemics in the United States since the 1964–65 epidemic, and rubella vaccine quickly took its place among the ranks of venerable vaccines like those against diphtheria, polio, and smallpox: another example of the promise and power of vaccination to control epidemic disease; another case that followed the same vaccine narrative.

More Diseases, More Vaccines

The structure of the rubella story parallels the polio story, but the specifics differ, and in some important ways, rubella vaccination's history is radically different than polio's. The particular historical moment and the specific cultural and institutional context were crucial to the nature and scope of the response to rubella. By the end of the Second World War, the American medical landscape—like much of American social life—was much more hospitable to major health research efforts than it had been during the period when pertussis and diphtheria vaccines had been developed. Even during the depression-era Roosevelt administration, the federal government had begun to take an active role in both funding and conducting research into medical and public health issues. When the Great Depression ended, the United States emerged as a world leader in most areas, including medicine and preventive health.

During the 1940s, innovations in production, spurred by the war effort, had made penicillin into a viable treatment for a wide variety of infections—it had become the new wonder drug, supplanting sulfa drugs and vaccines as the most impressive and far-reaching intervention against disease (Long 1949). As part of the war effort, direct federal allocations had funded the development of penicillin and research into a vaccine against measles. This established the federal government as a major player in health research, though private (and state and local government) groups still had an important role in vaccine initiatives, particularly in the case of polio. The rise of federal spending that had begun under Roosevelt and accelerated during World War Two continued to increase in the 1950s, and was crucial to the expansion of state and municipal public health departments, like those that had spearheaded the earlier vaccines. As the availability of funding increased, vaccine efforts also became less idiosyncratic, and more closely driven by the priorities of funding institutions, whether private or public. This new context also facilitated faster development. Funders, whether public or private, had broad social goals ("eliminate polio," "prevent the next rubella epidemic"), and they sponsored researchers, who—as in our current research model—would apply for funds to be used for specific initiatives that spoke to those goals. This was an important change from a time when research priorities had been largely set by individual researchers (like Pasteur), labs (like those in New York and Michigan), or even laboratory leaders (like Park) who would then seek support where they could find it.

The 1940s saw existing vaccines against diphtheria and pertussis receive AMA certification and enjoy increasingly widespread use (Felton and Willard 1944). Other vaccines, against tetanus, yellow fever, typhus, polio, and measles, underwent slow but active development through the 1940s (Plotkin and Orenstein 2004). Compared to these vaccine initiatives (in terms of the speed of accomplishments and the consensus around plans for use), the rubella vaccine efforts of the late 1960s were amazingly quick and unproblematic. The rubella vaccine research effort, certainly, seemed to exemplify the institutional maturation of the vaccine development process. The speed and efficiency of the rubella vaccine effort was partly due to the institutional factors described above, but it seems doubtful whether the anti-rubella campaign would have been so successful without the cultural experience of the Salk polio vaccine.

National publicity around the Salk polio vaccine trials reinforced the cultural story of vaccines that had been established among health professionals with diphtheria vaccine, so that by the mid-1960s, when the rubella epidemic hit, the vaccine narrative had taken hold in the general population. The expectation that scientists would discover a vaccine to protect against rubella-induced birth defects closely followed the story of polio vaccination, even though the institutions of vaccine development for rubella were vastly different than for Salk's research in the early 1950s.

Unlike the rubella vaccine effort, which was funded largely by the federal government, the work of the private National Foundation for Infantile Paralysis (NFIP; later known as the "March of Dimes"[2]) was crucial to raising the public profile of polio, as well as the money used to research and develop the Salk vaccine. After the success of the polio vaccine trials, the NFIP, which had been established by Franklin Roosevelt in the 1920s as the Warm Springs Foundation, was joined—and quickly supplanted—by the growing federal health bureaucracy, major research institutions, and universities in efforts to develop vaccines.

The broad institutionalization of health research practices reinforced more than laboratory methods and funding streams; it also regularized associated practices. For the purposes of clinical testing, researchers and funders recognized that vaccines had certain risks and they generally applied the "lesser harms" standard to evaluate whether it was even possible to test vaccine candidates. A vaccine had to compare favorably to the risks of the disease itself, and some polio vaccine candidates that came under consideration during the 1930s were withdrawn because of concerns about their safety during testing[3] (Halpern 2004). When an authoritative 1932 report on the status of research into the prevention, treatment, and cure of polio compared the risks of a polio vaccine to the risks associated with the disease, it concluded that "[i]n view of the low morbidity rate of poliomyelitis, widespread active immunization of human beings would probably never be attempted, even if a method of proved success were available" (ICSP 1932, 130). Absent a major public health crisis, polio researchers had relied on a relatively detached evaluation that weighed the risks of contracting the disease (and subsequent paralysis) against those associated with testing a potentially effective vaccine.[4]

Major events quickly and easily override even the most reasoned analyses of the empirical threat from a disease, and changes in the perception of the diseases meant that the calculation of risks and benefits began to compare the risks of the vaccine against worst-case scenarios for the disease. The polio and rubella epidemics were major events, indeed. Though the rate of paralysis from polio did not change between the 1932 evaluation and the 1950s, the perception of the danger posed by polio changed dramatically when, in 1952, the United States experienced a national polio epidemic, with more than 57,000 recorded cases (Paul 1971). By then there had been incremental improvements in knowledge and techniques for contending with polio. Following the successful model established by the anti-diphtheria vaccination campaign, researchers had been working to develop a preventive polio vaccine for use in a national vaccination program, and by the early 1950s, viable polio vaccine candidates were near ready to be tested.

The main response to the 1952 polio epidemic came not, as we might expect today, from the federal government, but from the NFIP, which had for many years been devoting resources to fund development of a preventive polio vaccine. The NFIP pressed for quick and very public vaccine trials. The rest, as they say, is history: by April of 1955, the Salk vaccine proved itself both effective and acceptably safe. The success of the Salk polio vaccine became part not only of medical and public health history, but also folk history. It marked a far more public recognition of the role of vaccination in disease prevention than anything since rabies vaccine in the mid-1880s, or perhaps even since the discovery of smallpox vaccine in the late 1790s. As the description of the response to and retelling of the polio vaccine story in the Introduction shows, the conquest of a frightening and widely dreaded disease (polio) by a preventive vaccine re-crystallized and reinforced the vaccine narrative: vaccines were capable of safely preventing children from contracting disease and, as the polio case suggested, mass vaccination of children held out the promise of defeating even the worst diseases.

Rubella vaccine seemed to fulfill the vaccine narrative from start to finish, and unproblematically. But congruence with the narrative's broad strokes—the development of effective vaccines to avert a feared epidemic—easily masks the special aspects of the rubella story. One important difference between the general narrative and rubella's case is that all three of the rubella vaccines that researchers had by 1969 developed to avert the anticipated epidemic had some acknowledged (though apparently mild) adverse effects associated with them. There were also important differences in the nature of the health problems that rubella caused, or rather the way rubella caused them. Although the birth defects associated with rubella were, like the worst consequences of polio, diphtheria or smallpox, frightening and dangerous, the attempt to prevent birth defects using vaccination opened a new area of disease prevention for vaccination. Rubella itself, after all, posed essentially no health threat at all to women—or anyone else—who caught the disease. The rubella vaccines deployed in the months before the anticipated epidemic at the beginning of the 1970s conferred no direct benefits on the people who got the shots. This development broadened vaccination's historical role beyond the idea of "complete control" of disease (by reducing morbidity) that the anti-diphtheria vaccination campaign had inaugurated. Diphtheria toxin-antitoxin had still offered a direct health benefit to vaccine recipients. In the rubella case, mass vaccination became a strategy to prevent a nominally harmless, if highly infectious, disease as a way to prevent *future* birth defects. The mass vaccination program begun just in time to avert the 1970–71 epidemic did not directly target women, some of whom might become pregnant and bear children with birth defects. Instead, American health policymakers decided to follow the polio (and diphtheria, and before that, smallpox) model and mass vaccinate children. The factors that led to this decision are complicated, and connected to the recent history of rubella, the attitudes and laws of the time, and the historical pattern of considering children the "normal" population to be vaccinated.

Before the national rubella epidemic, relatively few researchers paid any attention to rubella; there was certainly nothing like the NFIP to support and encourage research into rubella. Nevertheless, small and largely uncoordinated efforts to develop a rubella vaccine had been in the works from the 1950s, and the brief historical context that helped shape attitudes towards rubella and vaccination was crucial to the nature of the response to the 1964–65 epidemic.

Rubella and Abortion in the Pre-vaccine Period: 1941–1962

Following the 1941 discovery of its role in birth defects, researchers gave increasing attention to rubella as they tried to clarify the actual risks to the fetus associated with rubella during pregnancy and to find the causative microbe, with the hopes of proceeding swiftly to vaccine development. Consensus that rubella in a pregnant woman caused birth defects was neither immediate nor unanimous (Wesselhoff 1947), but the 1952 polio epidemic and the success of polio vaccine in the mid-1950s facilitated investigations that might lead to a rubella vaccine, both conceptually and in terms of the allocation of resources; the polio successes had brought vaccines unprecedented prominence in both the health professions and public consciousnesses (Katz 1974). Though during this time articles about rubella appeared only occasionally in the health professions journals, researchers very soon began to raise concerns beyond rubella's toll on newborn children born with CRS. They began to discuss rubella in terms of its relationship to abortion.

The connection between rubella and abortion was important because during the 1950s, abortion was illegal in the United States, with certain narrow exceptions. One exception was for medical reasons, including birth defects. This put medical physicians in the sometimes difficult position of being able to authorize legal abortions. Such abortions—called therapeutic abortions—had to be justified on medical grounds, and on that basis could bypass the legal prohibitions. Because rubella could cause CRS, infection with rubella during pregnancy became one of the accepted medical justifications for abortion; birth defects were the central medical feature of rubella, after all. In fact, rubella was one of the top indicators for a therapeutic abortion in the 1950s (Luker 1984).

The role of rubella in therapeutic abortion raised the stakes surrounding rubella, and complicated concerns about CRS and the need for a vaccine. Physicians who considered authorizing or performing therapeutic abortions would usually have to rely on an indirect diagnosis: they often had to listen to, believe, and then interpret after-the-fact testimony by women. Rubella's mildness, especially before researchers identified the virus in 1962, already made it difficult to verify cases, and a blood test for rubella infection did not become available until 1965 (Osmundsen 1965). Though there are no data to support it, it seems likely that many doctors would have been skeptical about testimony of having had rubella from young women requesting an abortion, considering reports about the general treatment of and attitudes towards women by the medical profession (e.g. Ehrenreich and English 1979; Corea 1985) and the AMA prohibition on abortion during that time. Doctors were quite clear about the possibility that rubella offered a justification for obtaining an otherwise illegal (and much less safe) abortion—a justification that was difficult to verify. One physician reviewing the state of knowledge about rubella in 1952 baldy asserted that "[t]here is a definite danger in the assumption that the patient who has rubella in the early weeks of gestation should have the pregnancy terminated. The diagnosis of rubella is sufficiently vague to be easily abused" (Tenney 1952). A better idea of the risk of CRS would help physicians with such decisions—and reduce the prospects for abuse of the therapeutic abortion option, but it remained unclear what that risk was.

Researchers and physicians pressed for better data in order to make a more informed decision about the risks of birth defects associated with rubella among pregnant women (e.g., Hill and Galloway 1949; Fox and Bortin 1952; NEJM 1952; Logan 1954). A simple answer was not forthcoming. Therapeutic abortions themselves could be a confounding factor in calculating precise CRS rates; some hospitals and clinics did not perform abortions, though a sizable proportion of institutions regularly performed therapeutic abortions without demur (Heferan and Lynch 1953; Horstmann et al. 1965). These problems fed uncertainties about the overall effects of rubella, including the rubella morbidity rate (which was difficult to measure directly because of the mild symptoms), the "real" rate of CRS among pregnant women exposed to rubella, and the importance of rubella as an issue for therapeutic abortions. In fact, there was a general paucity of hard data on the incidence of rubella, and therefore the rate at which CRS occurred. One study in 1957 found the rate of CRS among pregnant women exposed to rubella to be 9.7 percent, and possibly as low as 7 percent or even 1.9 percent, depending on how the birth defects were considered (Greenberg, Pellitteri and Barton 1957). Eight years later, estimated CRS rates ranged as high as 20 percent or 50 percent (NYT 1965a; Osmundsen 1965). Even so, some researchers' call for a rubella vaccine went beyond the implicit argument that birth defects needed to be prevented and that therapeutic abortions complicated efforts to understand the relationship between rubella and CRS. For these health professionals, a rubella vaccine was also necessary to reduce the number of rubella-associated abortions—to remove the medical loophole for abortion—irrespective of any data-gathering problems such abortions exacerbated.

The issue of the relationship between medical practice and abortion in an interesting one, though its complexities are beyond the scope of this analysis.[5] Historical and traditional foundations certainly existed for doctors' objections to women using a rubella diagnosis to obtain otherwise illegal abortions. Some researchers were outspoken about their opposition to medical complicity in therapeutic abortions, their argument was simultaneously against abortion and for a rubella vaccine: "Therapeutic abortion is . . . a direct violation of the fundamental ideals and traditions of medical practice" (Hefernan and Lynch 1953). Abortions performed on the pretext, rather than the actuality, of illness violated the law, and both professional and historical traditions militated against doctors performing abortions: the AMA had stood firmly in opposition to abortion since 1859 (Luker 1984) and the classical Hippocratic Oath includes the promise that "I will not . . . give a woman means to procure an abortion" (Porter 1996, 59). The idea that women might use the medical profession to skirt abortion law also challenged the power relationships between women and their doctors. Of course, with strict anti-abortion laws in place in every state, women might very well have sought to use rubella to obtain a "legal" and certainly safer therapeutic abortion without ever having contracted rubella.

This meant that abortion and the social place of women in American society, including women's role with respect to medical and public health policies and institutions, became central to the ways in which rubella became understood by health professionals. This was particularly true for doctors, who were the primary point of contact for pregnant women, and were the only people authorized to perform legal abortions. While the medical profession in the 1950s had nominally reached a broad consensus about abortion—officially abortion was forbidden, though there were exceptions, like for rubella—there was wide variation in how strictly the rules were applied, and individual doctors or hospitals were free to set their own policies.[6] As some key comments about rubella vaccine suggest, the health professions were primarily concerned with clarifying the epidemiology of the disease and scientific interventions that might eliminate the controversies associated with rubella. Vaccination against rubella offered to solve these problems.

In 1952, the editors of the *New England Journal of Medicine* voiced their concerns that alarmist estimates about the rate of birth defects caused by rubella among pregnant women could pose social and psychological problems for women. They asserted that "the solution to the problem is simple—for young girls to 'get the disease and get it over with' before they undertake the responsibilities of marriage and motherhood" (NEJM 1952, 132). An effective preventive rubella vaccine would serve the same function as contracting a case of rubella; it would confer life-long immunity. It could also "protect" women from (concerns about) having children with birth defects and indirectly help them fulfill their normative social roles as women. Even feminist critics acknowledged the power of such expectations for women's lives (e.g. Friedan 1963), but the idea that vaccines could or should help enforce aspects of women's roles as wives and mothers was an entirely new role for vaccines (though not for American medicine). Strangely, this was also not seen as a particularly radical use for vaccines. By this time, vaccines had become, like antibiotics, a powerful tool in the medical toolkit available to doctors and public health institutions. What had been an innovative intervention to prevent deadly epidemics had become incorporated into standard operating procedures.

The distinction between preventing birth defects (protecting the health of newborns) and preventing women from getting "unauthorized" abortions through a legal loophole designed to prevent birth defects became blurred when it came to the idea of a rubella vaccine. In both cases, a preventive vaccine appeared to clear the controversy and eliminate the problems. An effective vaccine would eliminate CRS birth defects (its primary purpose). By eliminating CRS, the issue of rubella-based therapeutic abortions would become moot. This ratio-nale stretched the utility of vaccines far beyond its traditional goal of preventing deadly epidemics. A rubella vaccine would do more than just prevent birth defects and save doctors from being asked to provide "dubious" therapeutic abortions. It would also, the professional dis-course suggests, protect women by making it easier for them to fulfill their roles in American culture.

The idea that doctors would protect women by developing a rubella vaccine transposed the benefits of the vaccine back onto the people who would likely receive the vaccine (women), even though rubella was not a threat to women's health. Although a successful rubella vaccine would, ideally, solve the problem of CRS, the focus on issues of abortion and "the responsibilities of marriage and motherhood" suggests the changed level of cultural acceptance for vaccines. In discussions about the search for a rubella vaccine, the desire to prevent birth defects became increasingly conflated with the idea of reducing or preventing the abuse of the thera-peutic abortion option and the desire to "protect" women by developing a vaccine. Rubella had at this point in its history never reached epidemic levels, had a mortality rate estimated at zero and the native rate of CRS resulting from rubella remained unclear, and perhaps unknowable.

The need to arrive at a reliable rate of rubella-related birth defects, to clarify the role of rubella in therapeutic abortion, and the sense that women, as child-bearers, needed protection against rubella for their own good, dovetailed neatly into a comprehensive argument for developing a rubella vaccine, to be used as part of a mass vaccination campaign. Research efforts continued at a steady but unremarkable pace through the 1950s, and in 1962 culminated in two independently published papers reporting isolation of the virus that causes rubella (Weller and Neva 1962; Parkman, Buescher, and Artenstein 1962). With the identifi-cation of the culpable germ completed by 1962, and a social imperative to justify the development of a vaccine at hand, it was time to proceed to the next chapter in the narrative: the development of an effective vac-cine, followed by mass vaccination and the eradication of rubella.

Vaccine Development: 1962–1970

The advent of the 1964–65 epidemic led to a rapid acceleration of the rubella vaccine project, as the larger medical research community and the general public turned their attention to developing a rubella vac-cine; the epidemic converted rubella from a relatively esoteric disease that had little currency outside medical journals into national news and a top priority. The short interlude between discovery of the rubella virus in 1962 and realization that a major epidemic was in full swing in 1964 did not see many important developments in rubella research, nor did it evidence any changes in the issues and attitudes that surrounded the disease and CRS.

The new and pressing problem of a CRS epidemic sidelined many of the issues about abortion that had been so prominent in professional discussions about rubella vaccine before 1964. Nevertheless, the fact that whether a child was born with CRS resulted from a woman's health status during the first trimester—a time when she might not even know she was pregnant—continued to be important for the ways in which the rubella vaccine candidates were formulated, tested, and ultimately deployed. That is, this was a vaccine that had as its ultimate target women who might become pregnant. Unlike any previous or subsequent vaccine, it did not confer any direct health benefits to the vaccine recipient. A case of rubella remained as innocuous as ever to the person who contracted it. And valid and verifiable rates of CRS remained uncertain.

In 1965 and 1969, international symposia on rubella and rubella immunization were held, and by the end of the decade three credible candidate vaccines were before the United States Food and Drug Administration (FDA) for approval and licensure. Though plans were proceeding quickly with development and use of these vaccines, uncertainty persisted about the rate of CRS resulting from rubella infection during pregnancy. Early estimates, based on very small studies, had placed the CRS rate as high as one in two (Green, Balsamo, et al. 1965; Schiff, Smith, et al. 1965) or as low as one in twenty (Greenberg, Pellitteri, and Barton 1957), but such estimates were, by the time mass vaccination began, generally recognized as unreliable (Dudgeon 1969). One of the problems with narrowing down the actual incidence of CRS, ironically, was "the relatively low incidence of rubella in women of child bearing age" (Cockburn 1969, 115) since the recent epidemic.

The rubella symposia concentrated on the immediate objective of developing the techniques and preparations involved in the production of effective vaccines; these were, after all, professional research meetings in which researchers reported their laboratory and clinical findings to their peers engaged in the same project. It is therefore no surprise that the discourse did not expend a lot of space (or energy) on justifications for what must have seemed an obvious project: to develop a vaccine capable of scotching a feared (and rapidly approaching) epidemic. Still, a reading of the symposia proceedings reveals concerns beyond the impending epidemic, linked to earlier considerations about abortion and women's roles. One of these was the call to create a vaccine to reduce or prevent "fetal wastage" associated with rubella, and the other was an increasing blurring of the distinction about who benefited from vaccination. Symposia papers repeatedly characterized women and fetuses—rather than newborns—as almost interchangeable beneficiaries of the anticipated rubella vaccine.

The connection between birth defects and fetuses is clear and direct—when a pregnant woman contracts rubella during the first trimester, the virus does little or nothing with respect to the woman, but can affect the fetus. This, in turn, can lead to congenital birth defects—to CRS. Rubella conference participants broadly recognized that CRS represented "by far the major problem of rubella as a disease" yet made regular reference to the 1964 epidemic and "its toll of many thousand cases of fetal wastage" (Prinzie et al. 1969, 172). This is not a comment about birth defects; it is not about children born with congenital deafness or children born at all. The phrase "fetal wastage" refers to spontaneous and induced abortion, and indicates the loss of fetuses before the pregnancy has been brought to term. Such a characterization of the rubella problem makes an important distinction between children born with CRS and "fetal wastage." The theme of fetal wastage was, in turn, closely related to concerns about abortion:

> This tragic aspect [abortion, both spontaneous and induced] of the rubella problem has been generally overlooked in published reports. It calls for more intensified efforts to improve laboratory methods for confirming the diagnosis of rubella and to develop effective measures for preventing infection. (Siegel and Peress 1966, 252–53)

An intentional abortion is, of course, very different than a spontaneous abortion (miscarriage) caused by disease, and preventing unwanted miscarriage (fostering healthy births) is a well-established medical and public health goal. However, the discursive continuum (or, perhaps, the "slippery slope") from protecting children from diseases, to prenatal prevention of birth defects, and from there to concerns about fetal wastage, is neither unproblematic nor uncontroversial, especially in light of concerns about the relationship between rubella and abortion. There was no dissent from the idea that "[r]ubella is a mild childhood disease for which vaccine would not be considered if it were not for its effect on the fetus in utero," (Detels 1969, 295) and that "[t]he aim in rubella is to prevent infection of the fetus" (Green et al. 1965, 362). Taken by themselves, such statements might mean little more than concern about preventing CRS.

In the context of other comments, however, it emerges that many of the concerns mentioned during the 1950s about the role of rubella in therapeutic abortions and the hope for a vaccine began in the mid-1960s to be expressed using the language of fetal wastage. For one researcher/ physician, the rubella-abortion connection was an "overwhelming personal tragedy. . . . [T]he extent of fetal wastage, and the expense accruing as a consequence of the recent rubella epidemic. . . . is sufficient to indict rubella as a major medical and social problem" (Weller 1965, 347). In fact, some researchers considered abortion, at the time still illegal and available to women only by way of the therapeutic loophole, an important social problem that a rubella vaccine could eliminate:

> Medicolegal and religious difficulties associated with therapeutic abortion and contraception are major facets of the rubella problem which can only be fully overcome by the use, early in life, of an efficient vaccine. Perhaps this will not receive universal acclaim as undoubtedly rubella has been the convenient scapegoat to terminate the embarrassment of many social mésalliances. (Forbes 1969, 9)

A preventive rubella vaccine, then, would not only reduce or prevent CRS, but help reduce the number of abortions.

Options other than vaccination, such as continuing the policy of therapeutic abortion, facilitated and informed by viral screening (a test had been available since 1965) received no attention at the rubella symposia. Viral screening for adult women was proposed only to remove the "legal and emotional consequences" involved in needlessly immunizing women (Karzon 1969, 386). The overriding consensus was that a preventive rubella vaccine would be safe and effective, and with high compliance rates such a vaccine could be a scientific solution to deal effectively with the "social problems" associated with rubella. This American approach contrasted with the British response; of course, Britain had not had a national epidemic, and also had a different cultural attitude towards vaccines (Baker 2000). During closing statements at the 1969 rubella symposium in Bethesda, Maryland, Dr. Frank T. Perkins, from the National Institute for Medical Research in London, England, commented that there had "been no official plans put forward for immunization against rubella in the United Kingdom," but that if there were they would likely begin with women likely to become pregnant who had "no circulating rubella antibody." Next, they would consider teenaged girls likely to become pregnant, and only then would rubella vaccine be "offered to the children to break the chain of transmission of the virus" (Perkins 1969, 383). In contrast, Americans planned to proceed with opposite prioritization: first mass immunization of children followed by "highly selective immunization of women in the childbearing period on an individual basis" (Karzon 1969, 384).

The task of preventing rubella from causing birth defects is a scientific, medical, and public health problem, with the obvious benefit of reducing birth defects for women who want to bear children. Many of the print discussions about vaccinating and protecting women glossed over this qualification, however, and treated *all* women as eventual mothers, and therefore applied the rationale of mass vaccination with a twist: researchers talked about prospective rubella vaccines as if they would protect women from disease, which was technically accurate, but from a disease entirely unimportant to the health of the women themselves. Indeed, the use of language at the rubella symposia shows a pattern of mentioning women as stand-ins for the fetuses they might someday bear: "The public interest in preventing rubella is related to the pregnant woman. How to protect women of child-bearing age is the main problem" (Murray 1969, 336). This has a natural kind of double-meaning: protection of women of childbearing age from the rubella virus using vaccines and/or herd immunity, but also protection of women from having children with birth defects and rubella-justified abortions. Women were considered the beneficiaries of rubella vaccine not because they would obtain immunity to the disease (which was harmless to them), but because they could then bear children without the fear or actuality of birth defects. Physicians repeatedly discussed women as the "target group"—the actual and final object of rubella vaccine (e.g., Karzon 1969, 384). The transposition, however, of woman and fetuses as the beneficiaries of vaccine use is difficult to construe as incidental. The comparison to the British plan supports this interpretation. These researchers appear to have thought of women as discursive surrogates for the fetuses they might someday carry.

Conferring authority on this view—and contrary to the idea that vaccines accomplish the goal of preventing disease by creating herd immunity—the U. S. Public Health Service's Advisory Committee on Immunization Practices suggested that men should not realistically be considered as recipients of the vaccine (PHSACIP 1969). Though the ACIP mentioned the possibility that "certain male adults, such as young fathers be allotted high priority on the basis of the fact that they may play a role in introducing virus into their household" (Karzon 1969, 385), such plans were never brought to fruition. Another researcher explicated the logic of not vaccinating men, explaining that "since the [rubella] vaccine offers virtually nothing to males, we can anticipate practical problems in inducing them to be vaccinated" (Beasley 1970, 158). This makes it clear that justifications for rubella vaccination de-emphasized herd immunity and instead viewed women as direct beneficiaries of a rubella vaccine. One result was the sense that cost-benefit calculations measured any risks associated with the vaccine itself against "real" benefits to the girls and women who would receive rubella vaccine.

Any vaccine contains risks and benefits. The promised (and publicly acknowledged) benefits of an effective rubella vaccine would be averting the 1970–71 epidemic, reduction in birth defects, and eventual eradication of the disease that could cause such birth defects. Other benefits that were apparently important to at least some researchers included elimination of the rubella-based justification for therapeutic abortion, reduced "fetal wastage," and protection for women to have children without fear of CRS. The risks of a prospective rubella vaccine were, according to the narrative, expected to be negligible, but even the safety of rubella vaccine was not so simple.

The Safety of Rubella Vaccine

Vaccines can be unsafe in a number of different ways. They can cause the disease against which they were designed to protect. This happened in the 1950s when a batch of Salk polio vaccine had been incompletely "killed," causing some recipients to contract paralytic polio, some of whom died from the polio that had been introduced as part of the vaccine. Vaccines can also turn people into carriers of the disease, without causing the disease. This was one of the problems with smallpox *inoculation*: it appeared to confer increased ability to survive an epidemic, but often made the recipient of inoculation a carrier—capable of spreading smallpox despite personal resistance to it (one of the advantages that smallpox *vaccination* had over inoculation was that cowpox never created smallpox carriers; it was also a lot safer: smallpox inoculation also sometimes gave the recipient smallpox). The third main category of problems with vaccination is called adverse effects. These are negative consequences that may or may not be directly related to the disease against which the vaccine is designed to confer protection, but which recipients experience as a result of vaccination.

In the research leading up to the development of rubella vaccine candidates in the late 1960s, there was little concern about giving recipients a case of rubella because the disease itself is so benign. The only exception to this was when the recipient was a pregnant woman, in which case a vaccine that unintentionally infected a pregnant recipient with rubella might cause CRS in the fetus, the very problem the vaccine was designed to prevent. There was considerable concern about creating rubella carriers, because although such individuals might themselves enjoy increased resistance to infection with rubella, their ability to spread the disease would contribute to the problem of increased rubella transmission, rather than reduce it; such a situation would "endanger pregnant women" (Plotkin, Cornfield, and Ingalls 1965, 388).

There were also concerns about adverse effects from rubella vaccines. Even before information about the connection between rubella and birth defects, researchers had some idea that there was a relationship between rubella and joint pain (Simpson 1940). Arthritis-like joint pain turned out to be an adverse effect of rubella vaccines, as well (Dudgeon, Marshall, and Peckham 1969). As one group of researchers encapsulated the purposes of a rubella vaccine, "direct protection of women [of child-bearing age] by rubella immunization would be highly desirable. . . . Although the arthritogenic properties of currently available vaccines are unpleasant, they appear to be as transient as those associated with unat-tenuated (natural) infection" (Cooper et al. 1969, 225). The appearance of these symptoms was coupled with the sex of the recipient, as it seemed that "[t]he occurrence of transient rubella-like symptoms after vaccina-tion is limited almost entirely to women" (Meyer 1969, 395).

Ultimately, concerns about adverse effects of rubella vaccines were noted but deemed acceptable. This was not a capricious decision, but one that grew out of a risk calculation that clearly prioritized the pur-poses of the vaccines: the discussions centered on protecting women as potential carriers of fetuses. One group of researchers noted that "[i]n considering the potential safety of a live rubella vaccine, perhaps our chief concern focuses on the fetus" (Meyer et al. 1968, 653–54).

By 1969, reports of adverse effects on women began to receive more direct acknowledgment, though the new information did not alter the evaluation of vaccine use. At the 1969 rubella vaccine conference in Bethesda, Maryland, two out of sixty-four papers presented dealt explicitly with adverse effects of rubella vaccine on women. They bear extensive quotation because they reveal attitudes about the importance of adverse effects, though the adverse effects appear to be relatively mild. The first was a study done on women vaccinated just after having given birth, but focused almost entirely on the vaccine's effects on fetuses:

> At the present time we do not know whether attenuated rubella vi-rus strains completely lack teratogenic potential [the ability to cause birth defects], and it is important to avoid administering rubella vac-cine during pregnancy. . . . Rubella vaccine could probably be admin-istered to women receiving contraceptives. . . . In the first nine vac-cinees arthralgia was not reported, but at that time we were unaware of that complication and no specific question was asked concerning

arthralgia. In 23 mothers which seroconverted [as the result of vaccination with HPV-77] specific questions relating to stiffness, joint symptoms and pains were asked. One case of arthralgia was reported: pain appeared in the knees five days after vaccination, lasted three weeks without local inflammation, and disappeared without treatment. It is difficult to say if this case was vaccine-related. . . . in comparison with observations of others, it seems that in this study with HPV-77 the incidence of arthralgia is low. (Boué, Papiernick-Berkhauer, and Lévy-Thierry 1969, 233)

The second article reported a study that compared the effects of two different vaccine candidates, "in adult women in an open field trial to compare vaccine effectiveness in stimulating antibody production and in relative frequencies of associated reactions." Its authors found that

Arthritic symptoms involving knees, wrists, or fingers were the most frequent manifestation of reaction. Three women [out of twelve] in each [vaccine] group had mild, transient arthritis which seldom lasted more than 24 hours and caused no appreciable disability. A fourth woman in the group receiving $HPV_{77}DE_{5+IgG}$ developed on day 13 a morbilliform rash and sore throat, followed by marked arthritic pain and swelling of the wrists and fingers. She was moderately disabled for nearly one week despite aspirin therapy. Three other women receiving $HPV_{77}DE_{5+IgG}$ suffered minor episodes consisting of one or more of the following symptoms: headache, malaise, pharyngitis, or slight fever. . . . Both vaccine preparations were associated with arthritic manifestations in approximately one third of the volunteers, however, the Cendehill strain seemed to be more attenuated in this respect; arthritis was milder and of shorter duration. (Byrne et al. 1969, 236)

Other papers at the conference reported similar findings, but only incidentally. Together, they established a consensus that all the vaccine strains had adverse affects on women (usually in the nature of arthritis), to varying degrees, and that these effects were considered acceptable[7] (Farquar and Corretjer 1969). In one case, researchers decided not test a particular vaccine strain (the HPV-77 strain, described in the first excerpt, above) because "of our experience with the high incidence of joint symptoms" (Dudgeon, Marshall, and Peckham 1969, 239–40). Another (Cendehill) strain appeared to have fewer and less pronounced adverse affects than the other candidate vaccines (Gold, Prinzie, and McKee 1969). Clearly, researchers were sensitive to the need to reduce adverse effects for women, though they passed both the HP-77 and Cendehill vaccines as having acceptably low adverse effects on women. One researcher at the 1969 conference summed up the attitude towards adverse reactions resulting from vaccines in general: "In the course of development and use of a number of vaccines it was recognized that untoward reactions could occasionally occur, and the possibility was accepted" (Murray 1969, 336).

The evaluation of the nature of adverse effects was (and is) a comparative one, and rubella researchers used the "lesser harms" standard developed earlier in the twentieth century. This standard compares a vaccine's adverse effects to the risks of the disease (Halpern 2004). In the case of rubella vaccine, however, the direct effects of the disease were essentially nil. The blurred distinction between preventing "fetal wastage" and protecting women meant that instead of comparing the risk of arthritis from rubella vaccine for women who might receive it to the dangers of a case of rubella for those women, they essentially compared it to the dangers of a case of CRS (but without considering the rate of CRS among children born to women who had been exposed to rubella during pregnancy, as that remained unknown). Given that comparison, much more serious adverse effects than even the mildest ones discovered in the rubella vaccine strains approved for use by 1970 might be deemed acceptable.

It is important to bear in mind the particular historical point in time that rubella vaccines were developed. American medicine was enjoying what has since been recognized as an extended period of ascendance. During and immediately after this period, revelations about ethical abuses and improper conduct began to increase outside intervention into medical decision making and administration, and eroded medical autonomy, cultural status, and the public's confidence in medicine and the other health professions (Rothman 1991). Though the specific adverse effects reported in the health professions literature were of a relatively mild nature, the tone and attitude towards patients and research subjects during this period often favored the research enterprise over subjects' rights.[8]

Proponents of a rubella vaccine were quite explicit about their enthusiasm, as they enjoyed the benefits of the still-rising tide of public successes, of which rubella vaccination would become another chapter. The polio vaccine hero Albert Sabin commented at a roundtable discussion at the 1969 rubella symposium that only about one-fourth of the women who give birth every year "would be rubella-susceptible, but we could not identify these women unless we screened for antibody. Those without antibody are the ones who need vaccine, but as Dr. Karzon said, it might be simpler just to vaccinate them all" (Sabin 1969, 388). Even within the history of vaccines, there existed options that could have reduced risks to women, but they were discarded in favor of a narrative that held vaccines to be inherently beneficial to the vaccine recipient. Screening for susceptibility was an important basis for earlier vaccine campaigns like that of diphtheria, at a time when resources were comparatively scarce (Miller 1940), but in rubella the idea was never seriously entertained. Rather than vaccinate only those susceptible to rubella (those without natural immunity), which was the option under consideration in Britain, American rubella policy consistently advocated a blanket mass vaccination approach. Interestingly, deployment of rubella vaccine in the United States did not begin with women, but followed the pattern of the earlier diphtheria and polio stories, and began with boys and girls. That decision conformed to the narrative—vaccines were to protect children—and also fit into existing patterns of vaccine delivery and enforcement. Schools were the place where states monitored vaccination compliance, and in previous vaccine stories vaccines had been administered in order to protect children.

Questioning Rubella Vaccine Use, *Roe v. Wade*, the IOM Report, and After

The story of rubella vaccine ends—almost—with widespread vaccination of children to avert the 1970–71 epidemic. There have been no more rubella epidemics, and no major outbreaks of CRS. The decision to vaccinate children against rubella stemmed from the same rationale as for earlier childhood vaccination programs: to establish herd immunity for the general population by creating an immune population of school-age children. Though the goal with rubella vaccination was specifically to protect women of childbearing years, the logic was the same as for childhood diseases like diphtheria, pertussis, and measles.

Despite the demonstrable success of rubella vaccination, comments critical of rubella vaccine policies began to emerge in the health professions literature soon after widespread vaccine use began. In a direct challenge to the accepted success of rubella vaccine policies, some questioned whether the absence of a 1970 epidemic could be traced directly to vaccine use, and whether CRS could be prevented through establishing herd immunity among children:

> Attempts to demonstrate "herd immunity" for rubella have been unconvincing. Also, some might argue that relatively little congenital rubella has been recognized since vaccination of children began in 1969. This reduction, however, can be accounted for by the infrequency of epidemics to congenital rubella syndrome, declining birth rates, and markedly increased availability of induced abortion. (Schoenbaum, Hyde, and Bartoshesky 1976, 309)

Both the issue of herd immunity and changes in abortion law are important for understanding the changing context for continuing rubella vaccination and the increasingly critical tone. The idea of building herd immunity among children was central to the rationale for vaccinating children against other childhood diseases (smallpox, diphtheria, pertussis, measles). Even before any widespread use of rubella vaccines, however, the U.S. Public Health Service Advisory Committee on Immunization Practices acknowledged that "by early adulthood, approximately 80% to 90% of individuals in the United States have serologic evidence of immunity" to rubella (PHSACIP 1969, 397). This means that only ten to twenty percent of adult women could then be expected to be vulnerable to rubella infection—not a surprise, given that rubella was historically endemic in the United States. Moreover, the consensus was that "only one in every 10 or 12 young women in the United States [in 1969] lacks rubella immunity"[9] (Meyer 1969, 395). If that is the case, it raises difficulties about assigning credit to rubella vaccine for averting the 1970–71 epidemic. The legalization of abortion further complicates the issues around rubella vaccination.

In 1973, the United States Supreme Court decision in *Roe v. Wade* struck down the laws restricting abortion throughout the United States. Because of the relationship between rubella diagnosis and access to abortion in the preceding decades, the decision became important for the purposes of understanding rubella and CRS: it changed the legal context. Legal abortion, available on demand, made the abortion-based arguments in favor of a vaccine moot. Rubella could no longer serve as a blind to obtain "illegitimate" therapeutic abortions. The abortion ruling also compounded the problems of accurate rubella and CRS reporting. Ease of access increased the number of legal abortions, which in turn magnified the problems of making accurate estimates of the rubella and CRS rates. Unless every aborted fetus were to be tested for evidence of rubella, a more accurante rate of CRS, and any chances of a good estimate of the rubella rate among pregnant women, would never be known. Even then, cases of spontaneous abortion, which often go unreported, would likely skew any estimates of the rubella and CRS rates.

The legalization of abortion in the United States also indirectly influenced the rubella discourse about pregnancy, birth defects, and fetuses. Although the earliest beginnings of the modern anti-abortion movement can be dated to the *Roe v. Wade* decision, the movement did not begin to take on a formal and coherent presence until the early 1980s. Much of the language of this movement, however, echoes the discussions about the need for a rubella vaccine. The legal changes brought about by *Roe v. Wade*, as well as the explicit discourse about freestanding "fetal rights," also meant that it became easier to talk about the rights of women as separate from the rights of fetuses. As the initial rubella mass vaccination was underway, researchers remarked on the unorthodox strategy that "[a]t the present, therefore, we are immunizing children in order to indirectly protect a third party, the fetus. This is a circuitous and unproven approach" (Neff and Carver 1970, 162). This comment recognized the novelty of using vaccination for an indirect purpose. A few years later, and shortly after the Supreme Court handed down *Roe v. Wade*, another researcher unpacked the nature of the third-party vaccination that distinguished the fetus from the "third party" who received the vaccine:

> unlike the other live virus vaccines, which were designed to protect the vaccinated individual against the consequences of a serious infection, the intent of rubella vaccine administered to children was to prevent disease in third parties once removed—the as yet unborn human fetuses. . . . unlike polio virus and yellow fever vaccines, which were essentially free of side effects, or measles vaccine, of which side effects were limited to transient fever, rubella vaccine-induced arthralgia or even arthritis [were of a different order of magnitude]. (Katz 1974, 615)

The second half of this excerpt reflects the increasing concern with adverse reactions to rubella vaccines in general, but also one strain in particular. Doctors increasingly reported "joint reactions" to the HPV-77 strain of rubella vaccine (mentioned above), and in 1973, the manufacturer withdrew it from use because of high rates of reactions in children (Preblud, Hinman, and Herrmann 1980; Hilleman 1992). But adverse reactions continued with the other rubella vaccine strains, particularly as vaccination programs were expanded to include women of childbearing age.

Adverse reactions were sufficient to warrant authoritative investigation. In 1991, the Institute of Medicine (IOM), the research arm of the National Academy of Sciences, published a study of the adverse effects of vaccination and concluded that rubella vaccine was causally implicated in both chronic and acute arthritis in women who had been vaccinated with it, especially as the age of vaccine recipients increased (Howson, Howe, and Fineberg 1991). The authors of the IOM report collaborated to summarize and publicize their results in widely read, high-status medical journals (Howson and Fineberg 1992a; Howson and Fineberg 1992b; Howson, Katz, Johnston, Jr., and Fineberg 1992). The IOM report was unquestionably authoritative, and it received praise for its objectivity and impartiality (Fulginiti 1992). Even so, there was no substantive policy response to the IOM report on the adverse effects of rubella vaccine. In fact, the same article that praised the IOM study for its impartiality argued for "additional scrutiny before acceptance" of the fact that rubella vaccine caused chronic and acute arthritis in women (Fulginiti 1992, 336). This response stands in stark contrast to the medical community's eager acceptance of the IOM's findings of "no evidence" or "insufficient evidence" for the adverse effects of pertussis (whooping cough) vaccine.

Despite wide publicity about the IOM findings within the health professions, in fact, rubella vaccination policy has not changed. Between 1985 to 1994, the American College of Physicians published three editions of their recommendations for adult vaccination during which warnings about the adverse effects of rubella vaccine for women became *less* emphatic (ACP 1985; ACP 1990; ACP 1994). Since publication of the IOM report findings, rubella vaccine recommendations in the United States have come increasingly to include adults. The issue is far from settled. Some subsequent research confirmed the IOM findings, particularly the increased adverse effects of rubella vaccine with increase in age (Davis et al. 1997), while other research found no evidence of any increased risk of new onset chronic arthropathies or neurologic conditions in women (Lin et al. 1996; Tingle et al. 1997). One article studying adverse effects reinforced the importance of continued rubella vaccination, repeating the injunction that "[p]arents need to be reminded that their child is susceptible to these diseases, that these diseases are preventable by reasonably safe and effective immunizations and that their child needs a series of vaccines" (Zimmerman, Kimmel, and Trauth 1996). Rubella vaccine, of course, offers small children something very different than polio or diphtheria vaccines do—if it offers them, as a class of people, anything at all.

Because rubella does not kill or even seriously sicken people who have it, there are unusual problems associated with promoting a rubella vaccine's acceptance and widespread use. Although it is probably easier to "sell" rubella vaccine on the merits of preventing birth defects to young women who are considering having children, that is precisely the population at higher risk for adverse effects. So the official and professional reticence to mention any adverse reactions to rubella vaccine, coupled with the cultural narrative that posits vaccines as our defense against deadly epidemic disease, has made for an unusual situation. Rubella vaccine has become simply another parallel story, alongside smallpox and polio, about the conquest of dangerous disease by vaccination.

The specifics of the disease, its effects, and the issues surrounding the vaccine cannot supersede the vaccine narrative.

The weak efforts by health institutions and experts to alert the public to the adverse effects make policy sense, as long as the professional consensus remains that rubella vaccination is necessary and important. But this is a problematic situation. For one thing, it might suggest a patronizing attitude towards vaccine recipients, by de-emphasizing some negative information that vaccine recipients should have in order to make informed decisions about vaccinations. This runs counter to current trends in the empowerment of patients and the recipients of health care, generally. When parents authorize mandatory vaccinations for their children (or when adults agree to be vaccinated voluntarily), they typically sign a consent form that includes information about all the known adverse effects. That kind of form, with its small print similar to the warnings found on many prescription medicines, is hardly a match for the power of a cultural narrative that we know, trust, and rely upon for our understanding of vaccines. Doctors, like nurses, are charged with maximizing vaccine compliance, and therefore typically represent vaccines as a positive, unalloyed good: they downplay any adverse effects and extol the importance of vaccination for the general public health and as part of the campaign to eradicate disease and its consequences (sickness, death, birth defects). Because of this, it is not clear that either the health professionals or most vaccine recipients "see" the problems with rubella vaccine as problems at all.

The idea that a vaccine is necessarily beneficial to its recipients is part of the narrative we tell about vaccination. The cultural narrative about vaccines describes them as a form of protection for the whole population from dangerous epidemic disease. Rubella vaccine does not fit this story—the direct beneficiaries of the vaccine are difficult to describe, yet discussions about rubella vaccine's purposes receive the same kind of description as polio or diphtheria vaccines. Extending the sense of vaccines' unequivocal usefulness to a case that does not fit the plot of the narrative particularly well shows an important aspect of narratives—they resist different interpretations of facts. Moreover, because they are not tied directly to particular facts, they are also highly resistant to facts that challenge the outline of the narrative. The way health professionals and researchers talk about rubella vaccination perpetuates the narrative that all vaccines protect recipients and the general population against epidemic disease and death, even though the facts in the rubella case are substantially different than for previous vaccines.

Rubella Vaccine's "Cultural Provenance"

Rubella vaccine was developed during what looks, from this point in history, like the heyday of vaccination in the United States. Though in many ways vaccination efforts are still going strong at the beginning of the twenty-first century, it was at mid-century that mass vaccination became the strikingly prominent and popular American public health initiative. Inaugurated by the publicity around the Salk polio vaccine, but carried forward through the 1970s with the kind of swift and effective response that rubella vaccine appeared to deliver in response to the projected CRS epidemic, vaccines promised high efficacy, safety, and the rational application of scientific medical knowledge to protect the general population.

The people who designed and developed rubella vaccine did so primarily to prevent birth defects. The evidence strongly supports the efficacy of the rubella vaccines developed during the 1960s: they could prevent infection with rubella by creating immunity in those who received the vaccine. The policy recommendations that came out of the professional discourse, however, suggest a different relationship: between the particular spirit of medicine and public health at the historical moment and the "cultural provenance" that vaccines had achieved by the late middle of the twentieth century. That is, the legitimacy imparted to vaccines by their meaning within the culture—their reputation based in the cultural narrative laid down during earlier campaigns against smallpox, diphtheria, and polio—was crucially important to the ways in which rubella vaccine has been and continues to be understood and used. The role of the narrative emerges in the decision to mass vaccinate children against a disease that was already endemic among them, and against which the vast majority of adults already were immune by the time they reached sexual maturity. This becomes clearer when we look at the ways in which rubella vaccine policies considered women its "targets" and the easy conflation of birth defects and "fetal wastage." The acknowledgement of adverse reactions for women and the decision to proceed anyway is part of—and plays an important part in—calculations of the "lesser harms" threshold. If we accept that there are concrete benefits to women (but not men) when they receive rubella vaccination, we are accepting their role as childbearing mothers as part of their medical identity.

It is not difficult to conclude that the prevention of birth defects is a legitimate goal of medical and public health policy. The largely unrecognized set of concerns, fraught with ethical and legal issues of individual rights (women vs. fetus), gender politics (the role of women as child bearers), and implicit (and sometimes explicit) opposition to "unnecessary" abortion, influenced the cost-benefit estimate. None of these issues is either inherently objective or scientific, and yet they have been central to both the professional and public understanding of rubella vaccine. Subsumed within the vaccine narrative, they received much less attention than they might otherwise have done.

Controversies surrounding vaccination have been exceedingly rare in the twentieth century, and there has been little public controversy about rubella vaccination. When groups and individuals critique vaccination policies, they often find themselves—and their claims—marginalized and discredited simply because they challenge the conventional wisdom. Publicity about particular medical failures or mistakes does occasionally result in a brief public exercise in muckraking, and reform sentiment. Cases in which there is a public perception of a breach in the public trust, such as the effects of thalidomide (Fine 1972), the Tuskegee syphilis study (Jones 1981), the excesses at Willowbrook (Rothman and Rothman 1984), or even the swine flu vaccine fiasco of the mid-1970s (Neustadt and Fineberg 1983), have worked in this way. They have generally not effected fundamental changes at the moment of public revelation, but rather have slowly contributed to the erosion of public confidence in medical decision making, ethics, and/or policies. The abiding salience of the vaccine narrative, however, seems to have insulated vaccination from these kinds of criticisms.

Narratives also function effectively within communities of experts. In the case of rubella vaccine, it is impossible to measure the extent to which researchers used purely medical criteria when evaluating costs and benefits associated with their research. Moral and social concerns infused and confounded both medical research and policy recommendations. The evidence of the historical record of print discussions within the health professions suggests that cultural and professional prejudices played an important role in the rubella vaccine research process. The direction of research in rubella vaccine was influenced by and rooted in social—rather than strictly medical or scientific—choices about women, fetuses, and the presumed role of vaccines in public health. The overmastering impetus for the creation and use of rubella vaccine was the prevention of unnecessary birth defects, but there was a strong initial component centering on opposition to abortion that elided the real and unprecedented ethical and epidemiological issues of third-party vaccination. There was also a tendency to ascribe only beneficial attributes to the use of vaccination as a practice.

Rubella vaccine remains an unglamorous vaccine, grouped almost anonymously into the trivalent MMR (measles, mumps, and rubella), and without any natural constituency to support or oppose it—except for established authorities and a strong cultural narrative, both of which support it. Although there has been mainstream scientific inquiry into rubella vaccines, complaints about adverse effects found publication only outside the mainstream—and even they were unable to manifest much support. With the growth of the Internet, contrary accounts have found voice—and it has become easier for non-professionals to find information about problems with rubella vaccination, including the IOM report itself as well as the professional journals that have contained the discourse analyzed here. Finding such authoritative sources, however, requires some determination. The most readily available Internet sources on vaccination can be found on anti-vaccination websites, which present seemingly authoritative accounts of dangers associated with a wide variety of vaccination programs. Their existence and influence, however, are largely passive—they are simply available for people who seek out such information. The only serious challenge in the late twentieth century to vaccine policies came from outside the medical establishment, and it concerned a venerable vaccine, against pertussis, that had, like rubella vaccine, authoritative evidence of adverse reactions, but much more serious ones.

3

Pertussis Vaccine
Resisting the Narrative

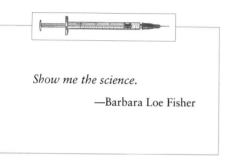

Show me the science.

—Barbara Loe Fisher

Challenging the Narrative

In April of 1982, the NBC television affiliate in Washington, D.C., broadcast an hour-long report called "DPT: Vaccine Roulette." It laid out a disturbing and to all appearances well-researched story about safety problems with pertussis vaccine. Organized like many other in-depth television reports on urgent social problems, the exposé interviewed medical experts on both sides of the question and used personal stories of children apparently affected by a common childhood vaccine to anchor and punctuate the program. With a somber tone throughout, the documentary represents in many ways a typical example of muckraking television journalism from the period: it attempts to present a balanced account of the pros and cons of a situation, while alerting viewers to unrealized dangers—in this case, dangers about pertussis vaccination. Though the program did not "take sides" in the controversy, it did publicly raise the question of whether pertussis vaccine caused significant neurological problems (Thompson and Nuell 1982). When parts were subsequently rebroadcast on NBC's nationally distributed "Today" show, this message reached a national audience (Fenishel 1983).

Still, the broadcast had a fundamentally critical tone, as in these introductory comments by the co-producer and host, Lea Thompson:

> For more than a year, [we've been] investigating the [pertussis portion of the DPT shot]. . . . What we have found are serious questions about the safety and efficacy of the shot. . . . Our objective . . . is to provide enough information so that there can be an informed discussion about this important subject that affects every single family in America. (Thompson and Nuell 1982)

The broadcast also gave both sides equal time. It portrayed representatives of the American Academy of Pediatrics, the Food and Drug Administration (FDA), and the Centers for Disease Control (CDC), who emphasized the safety and importance of pertussis vaccination, alongside physicians like Dr. Robert Mendelsohn, a Board Certified Illinois pediatrician and outspoken critic of vaccination and other medical practices (e.g. Mendelsohn 1979, 1981, 1984), and Dr. Gordon Stewart, Britain's most renowned opponent of mandatory vaccination. The focus on problems with the vaccine was clear.

By giving vaccine critics any airtime at all, let alone equal time, the broadcast violated one of the main proscriptions of the vaccine narrative: criticism of vaccines is itself dangerous. Moreover, it showed that even strong supporters of continued pertussis vaccine use implicitly acknowledged problems with the vaccine, which created a new and different kind of challenge to the narrative, in which critical ideas about vaccines could be spoken out-loud within the larger, popular culture.

In an interview midway through the program, John Robbins, of the Food and Drug Administration (FDA), explained the underlying concern about advertising even very rare adverse effects associated with pertussis vaccine, tacitly acknowledging that pertussis vaccine could and sometimes did cause serious problems in children who received it:

> I think if you as a parent brought your child to a doctor for a DPT shot and the doctor said to you, initially, "Well, I have to tell you, that some children who get this vaccine get brain damaged," there's no question what your reaction would be as a responsible parent: You would say, "I wish not to take this vaccine." But we do things as a community to protect each other. (John Robbins, in Thompson and Nuell 1982)

The nature of an exposé, after all, is not to ensure compliance with a policy, but to expose—such is investigative journalism's purpose and self-justification. In fulfilling these purposes, the broadcast came into direct conflict with the cultural narrative for vaccines. The relatively abstract vaccination bargain, in which individuals incur risk to accomplish a community benefit, is, it seems, vulnerable to challenge when people start looking at the bargain through a different lens, as the "DPT: Vaccine Roulette" broadcast did. Nevertheless, on the heels of public and successful vaccination campaigns against polio, measles, rubella, and mumps and, in 1977, the global eradication of smallpox, contention over pertussis vaccine safety seemed to catch the people and institutions that support vaccines entirely by surprise. Before this, Americans had little reason to question what they had been told about the safety and efficacy of childhood vaccines. Despite some very bad publicity in 1976 over the botched swine flu vaccination program (Neustadt and Fineberg 1983), vaccine compliance rates remained high, and most people had probably never heard of pertussis or its vaccine, and had given little thought to following the recommended schedule of vaccination as a routine part of protecting their children from dangerous diseases. The broadcast did not register any changes in vaccine compliance rates, and the most interesting thing about it was the discursive response it generated.

In fact, NBC's broadcast of "DPT: Vaccine Roulette" ignited a minor crisis in the public media, the health professions, and in the federal government. People who saw the broadcast began calling doctors, hospitals, and state officials, concerned about the dangers of pertussis vaccine. Newspapers editorialized about the broadcast and health professionals tried to reassure the public. In a May editorial extolling the achievements of vaccination, the *New York Times* implored researchers to ask "why the uncertainties it raises were not long ago resolved by careful study" (NYT 1982). The *New York Times* covered the news of the broadcast itself with only one article that stressed the minimal dangers of pertussis vaccine, while painting a frighteningly graphic picture of the disease itself. The article refused to repeat the claims made in the TV program but cited medical authorities' outrage at the NBC broadcasts to the extent that "[i]f there is such a thing as journalistic malpractice, this was it" (Altman 1982). The implication was clear: vaccines were too important and too valuable to be undermined by what they took to be either irresponsible journalism or careless research.

Response within the health professions literature was extraordinary. *JAMA*, the official journal for the American Medical Association (AMA), ran a highly unusual seven-page "news" article chronicling the fallout from the broadcast and the nature of the medical profession's response to it. The immediate solution was to control the damage done by mobilizing authoritative spokespersons to publicize the value and safety of vaccines, and reassert professional prerogatives. Recognizing that a publicity end-run had been made around medical recommendations, the article reassured readers that "physicians who support continuing DPT immunization have been fairly successful in getting airtime, at least in some cities" (González 1982). In questioning the safety of pertussis vaccine, the broadcast also posed a threat to the prerogatives of professional expertise and judgment—something on which anti-pertussis activists would later focus very closely.

In further reaction to the uproar generated by the program, members of the United States Congress called for public hearings about pertussis vaccine and its effects. The hearings drew medical and research experts to testify about the safety of pertussis vaccine, and ultimately certified the vaccine as necessary and safe—no policy changes resulted directly from the hearings. But the congressional investigation had an entirely unforeseen outcome. Publicity about the broadcast and subsequent hearings drew people from around the United States to Washington, D.C., including and especially parents who had seen the documentary and believed their children had been adversely affected by pertussis vaccine.

In bringing together these previously solitary and widely distributed people, the congressional hearings did something far more profound and far-reaching than NBC had done in broadcasting a documentary critical of pertussis vaccine. The hearings unintentionally facilitated the formation of an organized social movement group composed of people who had personal concerns about the safety of pertussis vaccination, as well as concerns about the wisdom of mass vaccination in general. In short order, these people who knew someone (typically a family member) they believed to be the victim of pertussis vaccine formed a new organization, Dissatisfied Parents Together, (or DPT, for short—the same acronym as the trivalent vaccine against diphtheria, pertussis, and tetanus) which would become the leading American organization opposing pertussis (as well as other) vaccination policies and practices (Coulter and Fisher 1991).

Although the "DPT: Vaccine Roulette" broadcast did not pronounce conclusions one way or the other about pertussis vaccine's safety, and the immediate fallout did not formally alter the rules or criteria regarding the use of pertussis vaccine, it inaugurated new kinds of engagement with the vaccine narrative. "DPT: Vaccine Roulette" openly contravened one of the narrative's most effective devices, that anyone who criticizes vaccines becomes a villain, a new danger to the entire vaccination project to protect the public health. The shudder that went through the health professions literature confirms this, despite the lack of effect on compliance rates or pertussis morbidity. Second, by indirectly catalyzing the formation of Dissatisfied Parents Together, the NBC program helped create a dedicated group of otherwise average Americans who, because of their own personal experiences with vaccination, were ready to challenge the narrative of vaccines on a wide variety of levels. Unlike previous anti-vaccination movements, which had focused on the rights of individuals or opposition to science in general, these critics of vaccination maintained a fundamental faith in science. They began to argue against pertussis vaccine practices using both scientific evidence and compelling personal narratives. In this, they found surprisingly strong support in the peer review health professions literature itself.

Although reports about dangers of pertussis vaccine (including those reported in the "DPT: Vaccine Roulette") may have come as shock to the general public, such reports were not news to health professionals familiar with the disease or the particular vaccine then currently in use. The people who made up Dissatisfied Parents Together adapted social movement strategies in innovative ways to oppose a widely accepted practice that was supported not simply by institutions, scientific expertise, and public policy, but also a strongly established cultural narrative. Any understanding of the events and processes around pertussis vaccination since the early 1980s must begin, therefore, with the disease itself, and its vaccine.

Pertussis (Whooping Cough) and the Cultural Context

At the time of the formation of Dissatisfied Parents Together, pertussis had become much less common and far less dangerous than it had been in the early twentieth century, when researchers developed the first vaccines against it (briefly described in Chapter 1). Average Americans in the 1980s were also generally unfamiliar with its symptoms, dangers, how it spreads, or how to contend with it. It has always been difficult to diagnose pertussis during the early—and most infectious—period, because it is not until the third or fourth week that the characteristic "whoop" can be heard, and the disease identified (the whoop follows paroxysmal coughing: an audible gasp for air). Thus, it tends to spread before it can be recognized. Over the course of the twentieth century, pertussis mortality rates have dropped; from an age-adjusted death rate of 8.0 per 100,000 in 1900–04, rates fell to 6.6 in 1920–24, 2.0 in 1940–44, and by the mid-1960s the death rate effectively reached zero (Erhardt 1974). Between 1979 and 1997, the CDC attributed no more than two deaths per year to pertussis—maintaining the effective mortality rate of zero per 100,000 (CDC 2000). The reduction in pertussis in the United States has been attributed to mass vaccination, though the greatest declines preceded the widespread use of vaccine. In addition, pertussis has, since the practical development of antibiotics in the 1950s, been curable with a course of erythromycin, but only if administered prior to the onset of the whoop (Berkow 1982). Antibiotics are also useful as a short-term prophylaxis during an outbreak (von König 2005).

Early in its history, the whoop was the only way to diagnose pertussis, though its putative cures were numerous (Radbil 1943). In 1906 Bordet and Gengou (1906) identified a likely candidate for the causative microbe, and researchers began to be able to test for its presence in children. Up until the 1930s, various individual physicians, public health officials, and bacteriologists argued for the use of a preventive pertussis vaccine using a combination of clinical reports and larger-scale controlled comparisons (e.g., Goler 1917; Barenberg 1918; Madsen 1925), but as I argue in Chapter 1, changing criteria for proof (Warner 1992; Meldrum 1994; Marks 1997) and the absence of an institutional sponsor for pertussis vaccine slowed approval for a vaccine. In the late 1940s, and based on results appearing in the peer literature (Sauer 1933a, 1933b, 1935, 1937, 1939; Kendrick and Elderling 1935, 1939), the American Medical Association's Council on Pharmacy and Chemistry reported renewed faith in standardized pertussis vaccine dosages and administration (AAP 1944; Felton and Willard 1944). Likewise, the American Academy of Pediatrics began in the 1940s to include pertussis vaccination as part of their Red Book recommendations, which form the basis for decisions by the United States Public Health Service about preventive health policies (Cherry, Brunell, et al. 1988). This vaccine was a "whole cell" vaccine that used attenuated—not killed—pertussis bacteria to stimulate the immune systems of the recipients.

In the early 1940s, pertussis joined the already established diphtheria vaccine in a bivalent vaccine, and later tetanus was added. The new combination—diphtheria, pertussis, and tetanus—came to be known by its initials, DPT, and became part of the standard schedule of vaccinations for all children in the United States. By the late 1940s many localities already had laws in place requiring diphtheria vaccination, and, coming as it did in a three-for-one package, there was little need to mandate pertussis vaccination separately; piggy-backed on the diphtheria vaccine, associated immunization laws, and recommendations from physicians, pertussis vaccination achieved high levels of compliance. By the mid-twentieth century, consensus about pertussis vaccine within the health professions had set aside questions about safety. The consensus that pertussis vaccine was effective, safe, and necessary fit neatly into the vaccine narrative, despite significant evidence of some relatively rare but serious adverse effects.

Evidence of pertussis vaccine's safety was not entirely unequivocal; such evidence rarely is. Unlike for other approved vaccines, however, peer reviewed, scientifically accepted studies and clinical reports suggesting adverse reactions to pertussis vaccine sprinkled the health professions literature on vaccines through the 1940s (e.g., Madsen 1933; Byers and Moll 1948; Globus and Kohn 1949). The main problems had to do with neurological damage, sometimes leading to death. Researchers who reported problems with pertussis vaccine almost always mentioned their strong support for continued use of vaccine, usually comparing adverse reactions to full-blown cases of the disease. One typical study concluded, after describing cases of neurological damage following use of pertussis vaccine, that "[i]t would be foolhardy to deny children the benefits of a comparatively safe immunization such as pertussis vaccine, when pertussis has such high morbidity and mortality" (Brody and Sorly 1947, 1016). This pattern continued into the second half of the century, as reports continued to surface about adverse reactions to the vaccine coupled with advice to use it—and vaccines in general—anyway (e.g., Kulenkampff, Schwartzman, and Wilson 1974).

By the last third of the twentieth century, mass vaccination had become an accepted and highly valued fact of life in the United States and other advanced industrialized societies. Politicians and medical researchers routinely credit the reduction in infectious diseases to our reliance on the mass vaccination of children. Some sociologists and historians have cast doubt on these claims by analyzing mortality rates relative to the introduction of vaccines or other medical measures; though the vaccines did have an effect on mortality, most of the mortality declines preceded the use of vaccination (McKeown 1976; McKinlay and McKinlay 1977). There has been a minor controversy among scholars of medical history and sociology over these findings (Colgrove 2002), though the findings have had no specific consequences for medical practice or policy.

Furthermore, the question of vaccine safety has remained secondary to the issue of efficacy. The calculus to determine whether to use a vaccine (or other public health intervention) is ideally based on a something like the lesser harms standard that was used to guide vaccine research (Halpern 2004), and an attempt to balance both safety and efficacy. American researchers, however, have typically considered efficacy much more crucial—and given it much more attention—than safety (Baker 2000). This is at least in part because of the differences in the kinds of criteria used to determine the efficacy and safety of therapeutic drugs: efficacy standards emerge from general practice, expert evaluation, and through clinical studies—all of which transpire within the professional community. Efficacy is also relatively easy to measure: whether in clinical case studies or in controlled comparisons in a large population, a drug either cures or it doesn't; a vaccine either prevents disease or fails to. Concerns about drug safety, on the other hand, have historically been "induced by disaster" and typically develop as the result of interactions between researchers and public attitudes (Bodewitz, Buurma, and de Vries 1987). Efficacy remains the primary goal and therefore dominates the whole process; unless efficacy can be established, safety concerns become moot.

Consideration of safety is also much more difficult to standardize. Determinations of safety rely on the interpretation of complex complaints from patients and require careful follow-ups for indeterminate lengths of time with patients who—in the case of vaccines—are likely to be otherwise healthy and whose symptoms do not conform to a standard diagnosis. The pattern is, understandably, that complaints and problems about patient care or the use of drugs (whether preventive or therapeutic) tend to originate with patients, and patients are rarely part of either the research or policymaking process. This situation leaves it up to health professionals to decide how to differentiate symptoms caused by a recently administered drug from those caused by innumerable other causes. These considerations apply, if anything, more strongly to vaccines than to therapeutic drugs. Perhaps the most important difference between preventive and therapeutic drugs is that preventives are by definition used much more broadly (especially when mandated by law), and usually administered to otherwise healthy people. The assumption in vaccines is almost necessarily that "one prevention fits all"—something assumed less often about therapies, where clinical differences can indicate modifications of treatment. Thus, safety standards for preventives (vaccines) could logically be expected to be higher than for therapies (cures or treatments for existing disease), because they need to be safer for a broader range of people. Because of the historical emphasis on the prevention of epidemics, however, this logic has not applied. When trying to avert a deadly epidemic, the emphasis understandably remains on establishing efficacy, with safety measured in relative terms (against the threats posed by the epidemic), and therefore receiving much less attention.

By the early 1980s, with the threat of high mortality pertussis epidemics long past, publicity about pertussis vaccine's safety alarmed American medical and public health authorities not just because they feared a decline in pertussis vaccine compliance rates and attendant increases in pertussis cases, though that was certainly a concern, but also because they feared a falloff in compliance with other vaccination requirements. In a kind of "domino theory" of vaccine policy, there was enormous anxiety that "fear and doubts about one vaccine may also affect the acceptance rates of other, totally unrelated vaccines" (Dudgeon 1986). A challenge to any vaccine, this reaction suggests, implies a challenge also to all vaccines and the principle of vaccination. This reaction validates the idea that, at least tacitly, vaccine proponents realized that something more (or other) than simply "the facts" about vaccination was involved in acceptance of and compliance with mass vaccination practices and policies. The emergence of a new, albeit very small, movement opposed to pertussis vaccination caused particular alarm.

Who Opposes (Pertussis) Vaccination?

Just as we all know the story of vaccination (heroic discoveries that avert epidemic death and free us from worry by the safe and systematic administration of vaccines), we also know the characters in the narrative who oppose vaccines. The narrative tells us that such people reject the clear facts about vaccination—that vaccination works and is safe. They are also crackpots, in the sense of fringe types who oppose common-sense interventions, reject basic precautions, and challenge the kind of normative civil society we all want (e.g., Hofstadter 1964). Such people might as easily reject pasteurization, fluoridation, and seatbelts. They would typically reject science (and the associated rational thinking), and because of their paranoid style, pose a danger to themselves and the public health as they undermine the fabric of civilized, modern society. Within the story of the vaccine narrative, vaccine opponents are ignorant, at best.

Of course mainstream bacteriologists and medical researchers felt that anti-vaccine views were both misguided and dangerous. But in the nineteenth century, when allopaths (regular physicians) had not yet achieved their dominance of American medicine, and average people often trusted other traditions of medicine more than they trusted allopathy or bacteriology, the boundaries of acceptable discourse were more open and fluid. Many people preferred homeopathic or other "alternative" medicine, and those traditions' opposition to vaccines carried considerable weight. One result was that the issues of vaccine efficacy and safety became bound up with the professional competition between the ascendant allopaths and other medical practitioners. When the allopaths and bacteriologists came to dominate American medicine during the early decades of the twentieth century, their support for vaccines (by then the list for general use included only smallpox, rabies, and diphtheria vaccines) became an article of scientific faith: to oppose vaccines was to support "alternative" medicine—to support quackery (Kaufman, 1967; Colgrove 2004).

The politics of the medical profession aside, there were also opponents to vaccination who eschewed ideological, religious, or political associations, and objected on the basis of safety concerns. Many people, including some regular physicians, opposed early use of smallpox vaccine because they felt it was too dangerous or did not confer enough protection, but such objections rarely found an independent voice, and tended to be lumped together with "crackpot" opposition. Part of the inexorable logic of science is that its very basis lies in empirical evidence. Over time, opposition to vaccination came to imply a rejection of science, the progressive uses of innovation (mass vaccination consistently promises to rid everyone—irrespective of class—of disease), and modernity itself; opposing vaccines became, on its face, evidence of some kind of crackpotism.

Given this history, it is not surprising that anti-vaccinationism did not persist in any significant form very far into the twentieth century in the United States, and today only a small minority of Americans actively opposes the use of pertussis vaccine, and ever fewer conform to the narrative's stereotype of a vaccine opponent, who believes quackery and distrusts science. Many Americans, however, have become more skeptical about vaccination in general. As one researcher interested in boosting compliance rates found, most parents who have concerns about vaccines being unnatural and dangerous are not crackpots, as he put it, they "are not fringe types; far from it. Simply put there is a sizeable majority of middle America that is fearful that recommended vaccines may do their child more harm than good" (Marcuse 1991, 88). Of course most people do comply with vaccination requirements, but that "sizable majority" of families from "middle America" worries vaccine policymakers because it might be susceptible to alternative views on vaccines—to other stories about them.

Unlike the establishment of consensus within the health professions, which has its own normative requirements, consensus within the general population is generally not believed to depend on cool-headed evaluation of empirical scientific data. No one expects everyday Americans to read and understand the medical and scientific journals where the evidence of vaccine efficacy has been established. Health care professionals continue to emphasize ignorance as the basis for non-compliance with mass vaccination (Frenkel and Nielsen 2003), even though studies have found that non-compliance with vaccination programs is actually correlated to high levels of education and unrelated to "ignorance" about vaccination (Gust, Strine, et al. 2004; Maayan-Metzger, Kedem-Friedrich, and Kuint 2005).

With renewed opposition to pertussis vaccination in the early 1980s, "middle America" became the contested ground between authoritative medical institutions supporting mass vaccination and the small group of parents who constituted Dissatisfied Parents Together. Although mainstream social movements theory tells us that resources, cultural authority, access to the public media, and strong institutions are a recipe for success (Blumer 1969), the David and Goliath nature of the contest between a small determined group of activists and organized health professions meant that, in this case, the established authority had much more to lose, and was therefore in some ways more vulnerable. This is especially true considering that for vaccination advocates only complete cultural acceptance of vaccination, and extremely high compliance rates, could qualify as success.

A Different Kind of Challenge to Scientific Consensus

There is little authoritative dispute that most vaccines work—each vaccine confers protection for months, years, or a lifetime against a specific disease. From the early smallpox vaccine case studies presented by Edward Jenner in the 1790s to the public trials of Salk's polio vaccine in the 1950s, the empirical evidence on efficacy has spoken without equivocation: in an epidemic, vaccination confers life-saving protection. Since then, more sophisticated clinical trials and widespread vaccine use have convinced medical experts that vaccines can be highly effective preventives even in non-epidemic situations. These conclusions, however, have come out of the health professions—a community of experts—and have not automatically transferred to the general population. Populations rarely ask for a mass vaccination program to be implemented, though they sometimes clamor for help—for experts to produce a vaccine (as happened during the AIDS epidemic). More often, lay populations begin with some level of skepticism about scientific innovation, and only after the slow process of dissemination and what has come to be called "public relations" do innovations typically achieve acceptance in the general population. That happened for mass vaccination over a period of 160 years, primarily through the smallpox, diphtheria, and polio vaccine campaigns, with lesser-known vaccines benefiting by association. Ultimately, though, these innovations originated with a professional consensus among experts. Opposing experts in their own field is a difficult undertaking.

Although the movement that began in the early 1980s to oppose the scientific consensus about pertussis vaccine was by no means the first such movement, it introduced innovations into the conduct of oppositional anti-vaccine campaigns, and in many ways foreshadowed the more widely know and better studied successes of the AIDS activism movement that began later in the decade. Like AIDS activists, modern anti-pertussis vaccine activists relied on the motivation of their members stemming from personal relationships to the issue, but unlike many AIDS activists, the opponents to pertussis vaccine had no access to pre-existing networks or community structures. Anti-pertussis vaccine activists also inaugurated some new tools for opposing medicine and science. They strategically used mainstream scientific and medical evidence together with effective re-telling of the vaccine narrative from the perspective of a victim of adverse effects resulting from pertussis vaccination.

In most other respects, the anti-pertussis vaccine movement fits the conventional view of an oppositional social movement. The leaders of Dissatisfied Parents Together have been well educated, articulate, and from the middle class, like most activists in science-based movements (McCarthy and Zald 1973), and their ready ability to access the technical medical literature constitutes an important resource. Their willingness to embrace the logic and cultural provenance of scientific research, however, sets them apart from all previous anti-vaccination movements, and puts them within a very small group of collective action groups that has used similar strategies. Anti-pertussis vaccine activists felt betrayed and disenfranchised by the individuals and institutions they had trusted, and like many people suffering personal tragedies, they sought meaning and some kind of recognition and redress for their suffering (Kaplan 1997), but with an important ontological difference. As Barbara Loe Fisher, president of Dissatisfied Parents Together, put it, "If the science is well done, I'll be the first to line up with my kids. Show me the science" (Fisher 2000). Although there are important similarities between the anti-pertussis vaccine movement and other organized movements challenging accepted scientific programs, the anti-pertussis vaccine movement adds an interesting variation to our understanding of such movements as "anti-science."

Understanding Dissatisfied Parents Together's opposition to vaccination requires understanding the group not just in terms of vaccines, but also as a social movement. This movement's connection to science—rather than to morality, individual rights, or the public good—makes it possible to see contention about pertussis vaccine as a situation involving competing social movements (della Porta 1999) rather than issues about diffusion of technology (Hollingsworth, Hage, and Hanneman 1990) or opposition by crackpots (Hofstadter 1964). Though both "sides" use issues of morality, individual rights, and the public good to assert the validity of their positions, the largely common language of contention makes it a natural case to try to span the theoretical divisions between sociologists and historians interested in more relativist (Shapin

1992; Löwy 1992) or more objectivist (Moulin 1991; Mazumdar 1995) frames of analysis for understanding scientific controversies. That is, because Dissatisfied Parents Together used peer reviewed research as the cornerstone of its case against pertussis vaccine, the organization's positions were not so easily (or automatically) discredited. This forced both sides at least implicitly to acknowledge the contested narrative as a main field of battle.

What analyses exist about anti-vaccinationism as a social movement have typically assumed the modern movement to be "just another case" of opposition to science and technology over issues like control and public involvement (Nelkin 1992). The idea that opposition to vaccines would not be based on substantive issues about the vaccines dovetails neatly with the vaccine narrative—opponents must, at least at some level, be off-base. In opposing pertussis vaccine, for the first time vaccine critics used scientific arguments and within those arguments, restricted themselves to the language of objective science to challenge an established medical practice. This meant that the science itself was not in question; instead, the recourse to scientific evidence called into question the judgment of the researchers who had interpreted the science, and hence, their professional expertise. The focused assault on the conclusions of the experts based on a common corpus of data—the peer reviewed literature—forced the medical community to respond in a different way than it had to previous anti-vaccination movements.

In their publications and on the Dissatisfied Parents Together website, anyone interested in the scientific evidence about pertussis vaccine find citations to articles from journals like: *Acta Pediatrica Scandinavica, Archives of Disease in Childhood, British Medical Journal, Cellular Immunology, Journal of Pediatrics, JAMA, The Lancet, Medical Officer, Nature, Neurology, Neuropediatrics, New England Journal of Medicine, Pediatric Infectious Diseases,* and *Pediatrics.* The ability to quote research critical of pertussis vaccine safety from the *Journal of the American Medical Association,* the organ of the AMA, provides opponents access to the powerful cultural authority of modern, objective medical science. This, after all, is the foundation on which so much of the health professions' status rests: the authority of science itself.

But scientific communities have their own norms and rules, and don't easily allow outsiders to influence their processes. There are two main models for how science-based consensus is determined. The positivist model assumes that the quantitative methods of science in the service of convincing argument can approach some kind of "truth" and therefore operate outside the realm of power, influence, ideology, and prejudice. A more sociological model, in contrast, while unwilling to reject all aspects of positivism, recognizes the important role of structure, power, and ideology in the kinds of outcomes that are possible for scientific actors to consider. For the case of vaccines, and pertussis vaccine in particular, all of these factors feed into and are fed by the broader cultural narrative about vaccines, and how we, as a society, view and value them.

An example unrelated to vaccination makes it easier to see the modern anti-vaccination movement more clearly. In trying to understand the resilience of anti-fluoridation movements in the face of generally accepted scientific knowledge, sociologists generally ascribe anti-fluoridationists' impressive record of success (they have consistently blocked efforts to add fluoride to the drinking water in many otherwise progressive and science-friendly communities) to a kind of populist anti-scientism that mobilizes sectors of the general population by appealing to fears about government control (or of communism, etc.), opposition to interference with nature, or by positing a "conspiracy of experts," etc. (Crain, Katz, and Rosenthal 1969; McNeil 1985). A more nuanced sociological analysis of the history of fluoridation, by contrast, argues that the exemption of the products of science from sociological examination—assuming that the evaluation of science is the sole province of scientific experts—skews the analysis. Perhaps the focus of research on movements opposing organized science should not be limited to trying to understand, essentially, cases where crackpots may succeed (i.e., how the progress of science can fail). Rather, the obligation is to look to an examination of "the processes of scientific opinion formation" (Martin 1989, 72) to understand how competing ideas gain their currency and power in society.

This makes much more sense if we can acknowledge the extent to which narratives help structure our worldview. When the health professions community responded to the initial challenges about pertussis vaccine safety (or to other, earlier, challenges to mass vaccination), their arguments about the cost-benefit ratio reassured federal and state governments, which were ready and willing to accept their status as expert professionals. But among the general population, attempts to discredit Dissatisfied Parents Together as alarmist crackpots met an audience that was not so easily impressed by expert credentials, partly because the general (popular) acceptance of vaccines had never been based on a clear understanding of immunology or statistical epidemiology.[1] Americans have typically accepted vaccines, arguably, because they have accepted a cultural narrative that incorporates vaccination as a central theme in public health.

[97]

The struggle for power between the competing groups over pertussis vaccine began in the science-laden discourse about pertussis vaccine from health professions journals, though it quickly moved to other arenas. That shift did not serve the interests of pro-vaccine forces, though they ultimately prevailed (unlike nineteenth-century anti-vaccination groups, Dissatisfied Parents Together did not succeed in repealing any laws that mandated pertussis vaccine); it meant that vaccine opponents could use their own counter-stories to make their case against pertussis vaccine. This discursive change of venue happened because of the strategies and nature of Dissatisfied Parents Together.

Dissatisfied Parents Together/ The National Vaccine Information Center

Dissatisfied Parents Together and the National Vaccine Information Center (DPT/NVIC) are two aspects of the organization founded in 1982 with the stated goals of "gathering information about pertussis and the pertussis vaccine, getting that information out to parents, and finding ways to lessen pertussis-vaccine damage" (Coulter and Fisher 1991, 138). The NVIC is the non-profit arm of Dissatisfied Parents Together. Their organizational structure falls somewhere between those movement organizations that mobilize members and have a political goal and others, called "supportive organizations," that facilitate movement organizations' goals (Kriesi 1996). Dissatisfied Parents Together self-identifies as a service organization that responds to concerned parents and advises them, provides information generally, and acts as a "watch-dog" on pharmaceutical companies (Fisher 2000). It sees itself as performing an alternative but parallel kind of public service to the public that the mainstream public health institutions will not provide, though Dissatisfied Parents Together is obviously much smaller and less authoritative than the Public Health Service.

The organization's staff consists of a president, a director, and a handful of part-time office workers. All of the "office staff" (including the officers—who are also the co-founders), have personal investments in the anti-pertussis movement in the form of a family member or close friend believed to be vaccine-affected. From its beginnings as an all-volunteer organization of (mostly) mothers working out of their homes, DPT/NVIC has since become an organization with a national reach (Fisher 2000). In 2000, DPT/NVIC reported more than 30,000 members nationally, with an annual budget of around $700,000. Its income derives primarily from small contributions from members, with less than ten percent coming from the sale of books, literature, and in the form of direct grants from foundations. Dissatisfied Parents Together has an office (since 1994), a toll-free phone number, and an active and award-winning Internet website (Williams 2000). This formalized and increasingly institutionalized state of affairs is the result of a slow evolution from the organization's beginnings in the early 1980s.

Dissatisfied Parents Together's leaders describe their mission as being dedicated to public education about the dangers of pertussis (and other) vaccines, providing counseling to parents and grandparents, opposing the expansion of mandatory vaccination laws, and helping to guarantee financial compensation for serious reactions they attribute to use of the vaccine (Fisher 2000). They do not say that they advocate banning all vaccines or vaccinations, and in 2000 the NVIC inaugurated its own new funding initiative, "The Children's Fund for Hope and Healing," to provide funding for people who want to do high-quality scientific research into adverse vaccine reactions. Taken at face value, this kind of activity suggests a philosophy that makes them more like the AIDS organizations that have allied themselves with major research efforts than other historical movements opposed to vaccination, or even those opposed to medical or public health measures, generally. The organization's website, however, features a "memorial" to the victims of vaccination generally—whether from pertussis, anthrax, influenza, or other vaccines.

There is also a pervasive feeling of a moral crusade stemming from the sense of betrayal. As Dissatisfied Parents Together's leaders explained almost two decades of commitment: "We do this out of a passion for this work, for this mission" (Williams 2000). The mission is to save innocent children from unnecessary exposure to health risks. What higher moral claim on medical science can there be than young children's right to health? It is—not coincidentally—also the narrative claim that health professionals make for vaccine use. In this, as well, the modern anti-pertussis movement has used aspects of the vaccine narrative to gain entry into the public discussion about vaccine safety and usefulness.

However, their lack of professional status has largely excluded them from the institutionalized forums for discussions about medical and scientific evidence and the peer review literature, and—unlike AIDS activists—Dissatisfied Parents Together has not broken through the wall that separates credentialed experts from lay experts and other interested parties. So, despite their innovative use of science in opposition to science, the field on which modern anti-pertussis activists' challenge to pertussis vaccination has succeeded (to the extent it has) has often been in direct appeals to public opinion, in the legal system (through support for tort litigation), and in political lobbying (Heller 2005). Their use of science in these realms has been central to participation in negotiations with health professionals and policymakers on legal and policy issues, even if they have not limited themselves to scientific arguments.

Their pamphlets and publications cast their concerns in terms of individual vaccine recipients' health and safety, which are the same goals as vaccination programs themselves. In Dissatisfied Parents Together's view, vaccination is a public health policy designed by the medical profession, sanctioned by the federal government (through the Public Health Service, the Surgeon General, etc.), and enforced by individual state governments, which has caused not the promised unproblematic protection from disease, but tragic vaccine-related adverse reactions. *A Shot in the Dark: Why the "P" in the DPT Vaccination May Be Hazardous to Your Child's Health*, co-authored by one of the founders of Dissatisfied Parents Together, offers a quick summary of the case against pertussis vaccine:

> The following serious reactions to pertussis vaccine are documented in more than fifty years of scientific literature and many are mentioned in guidelines produced for doctors by the American Medical Association (AMA), the American Academy of Pediatrics (AAP), the Centers for Disease Control (CDC), and vaccine manufacturers: high fever (over 105°F); convulsions (with or without fever); unusual high-pitched screaming; persistent crying for more than three or more hours during which the child cannot be comforted; excessive somnolence (deep sleep from which the child can be awakened only with great difficulty); collapse (a sudden loss of consciousness); encephalopathy (brain damage); and death. (Coulter and Fisher 1991, 1–2)

Like their pamphlets, this quotation encapsulates the elements of the pertussis vaccine opposition position. The passage contends that pertussis vaccine has a wide range of dangerous side effects, and—significantly—that there is solid and authoritative scientific evidence for them. It is directed at non-scientist parents of children (note the layman's clarifications of terms like "somnolence" and "encephalopathy"). The purpose of publishing such a book is clearly to carry out the mandate of the organization—to "spread the word" about the dangers of pertussis immunization, gain new adherents, and therefore expand pressure on the very institutions and agencies mentioned in the quotation to end or restrict the use of pertussis vaccine. Their book also intersperses personal stories of tragedy with factual and historical explanations of the problems with pertussis vaccine; emotional appeals and moral outrage have from the beginning been part of the Dissatisfied Parents Together's strategy to change vaccination policies and practices. (Despite this, the book stands as an excellent resource for information about adverse effects of vaccines—it contains reference to much serious scholarship.) This double strategy accesses both the emotional shock value of images and personal stories of vaccine-damaged children, while it seeks to access the cultural clout and authority of scientific expertise.

Before 1982, opposition to pertussis vaccine existed in the United States, but only at an individual level, usually parents of children who believed that pertussis vaccine had injured their children. These people resorted to the court system, and Dissatisfied Parents Together continued to use the legal route as a way to leverage change in the institutions of pertussis vaccination. In these attempts, Dissatisfied Parents Together has not been without support from individual doctors who used their status to testify against pertussis vaccine and vaccines in general (e.g., Mendelsohn 1984); such activism typically costs doctors their credibility within professional circles. These medical—and therefore "elite"—opponents of pertussis vaccine allied themselves with their counterparts and recent predecessors in Britain, whose criticisms of pertussis vaccine had embroiled British medical institutions in controversy since the mid-1970s. For some time before the anti-pertussis movement began in the United States, British researchers and physicians had engaged in a spirited internal debate about the continuing value of pertussis vaccine.

Like the homemaker activists in Love Canal, Dissatisfied Parents Together members made up for their own lack of professional status by invoking objective studies in their attempts to use science to undermine the credibility of the medical establishment's pertussis policy (Kaplan 1997). Such information, available in the health professions literature to anyone who sought it, had not, by 1982, had any effect on vaccine policies or practices. Nor did an actual "accident" involving pertussis vaccine: in 1979, the U. S. government ordered the recall of more than 100,000 doses of diphtheria-pertussis-tetanus vaccine produced by Wyeth Laboratories after 4 babies in Tennessee died within 24 hours of receiving the injection (NYT 1979). Only with the NBC broadcast of "DPT: Vaccine Roulette" was there a crucial publicity crisis of the kind that has been shown to be of potentially great importance to issue-oriented social movements (McCarthy, Smith, and Zald 1996). Suddenly the pro-vaccination establishment had what Bodewitz et al. (1987) call a safety-related "disaster" with which they had to contend. The disaster was not based on the "real" event (the death of four children and the recall of vaccine doses), but on the discursive event—the narrative disaster—of the NBC television special. While the bad batch of vaccine endangered lives, and spoke directly to the safety of pertussis vaccine preparations, the television program threatened the dominance of the narrative, and was in that way a more potent threat to the cultural understanding of vaccines.

The track record of Dissatisfied Parents Together in American courts and legislative bodies shows that those venues are surprisingly open to the use of scientific evidence to establish facts or to cast doubt upon them. As was so often the case in the fluoridation controversies, this supports the idea that lay audiences are much more receptive to contrary scientific evidence than professional audiences (Jasanoff 1997; Faigman 2004). Despite the scientific community's pervasive ontological claim that its methods and very *raison d'être* are rooted in the premise of considering and evaluating contrary evidence (a theory can never be proved, only disproved), health professions scientists have remained highly resistant to considering claims once the professional consensus had established pertussis vaccine's safety. The corollary is that the rarefied discursive space of professional science appears highly intolerant of minority views or evidence that might disconfirm established modes of thinking. Consensus seems to trump debate.

The modern anti-pertussis vaccine movement remains motivated by the goal to protect children from serious, but unintended, reactions to the vaccine. The stated philosophy of Dissatisfied Parents Together looks to institutionalized science for authority:

> NVIC is working for wider recognition that well-designed, independent, on-going scientific investigation must be conducted to define the biological mechanism of vaccine injury and death and evaluate the chronic, long-term effects of multiple vaccination on individuals and the public health. (NVIC 1998)

This amounts to a call to re-evaluate the accepted conventions about vaccine safety. It asks health professionals to second-guess themselves and their own consensus, because the evidence on pertussis vaccine has already been presented, evaluated, and considered within the health professions community. But people opposed to pertussis vaccination also presented their own "data" for consideration.

In addition to citing reports published in the medical literature, Dissatisfied Parents Together has relied heavily on personal stories of vaccine-induced illness—presented as avoidable tragedy—to bolster their claims about vaccine's dangers. This sometimes looks like a blatant appeal to emotion, rather than to science. The language used, however, particularly in the longer descriptions, as in *A Shot in the Dark*, seems designed to resemble an anecdotal report on safety data. Though it is clearly not within the rhetorical discourse of late twentieth-century science—it more closely resembles early twentieth-century clinical reports—it might qualify as a kind of empirical scientific data collected by parents about their children's symptoms. It can be seen as an attempt to append data to the medical record (though it has a powerful emotional impact, as well). The mother of a one-year-old with a history of meningitis, after telling her doctor—before vaccination—that her daughter had recently had a cold infection, was in turn told, "I don't think it will be any problem." This selection follows:

> Leigh's mother remembers what happened after they got home. "A little more than an hour after Leigh had the shot, she started crying hard. Then she had violent explosions of gas. At the same time the site of her injection swelled up. It was a huge swollen area. Then she started screaming. She screamed for sixteen hours non-stop. Her scream sounded so painful, I thought she had meningitis again. She finally got a little sleep the next morning, but she literally cried for sixteen hours without stopping. After she woke up, she cried on and off for two more days and nights." Within the next few days, Leigh began clenching her fists, bending her elbows, and turning her arms inward to her body. She was no longer able to stretch her arms out in front of her or over to her side. She did not sit until she was twelve months old or try to crawl until she was fourteen months old. Now she is almost three and cannot talk. She has been diagnosed as mentally retarded. "A neurologist told me that, unless she had a grand mal seizure within twenty-four to forty-eight hours of the shot, they don't consider it a causal relationship." (Coulter and Fisher 1991, 132)

The description of immediate post-vaccination events by the child's mother, though clearly framed to convince the reader that the vaccine is responsible, is also what one might expect her to have said to a doctor. Yet it reads more like a clinical description of symptoms than the complaint from a distraught parent.

In appealing to the empirical nature of reports from parents, Dissatisfied Parents Together tried again to use medical institutions' own best weapon—the cultural authority of dispassionate empirical scientific (in this case clinical) evidence—to their own ends. The attempt to stay within the broad heuristic of modern medical science while incorporating highly emotional narratives about small children hearkens back to the kinds of individual clinical reports that modern population-based vaccination studies had displaced in the early decades of the century. In trying to reassert the importance of individual experiences, pertussis vaccine opponents insist that science can still be trusted, but that the judgments made about safety depend on the kind of scientific data used in the analysis, and the place of the individual in that analysis. In this way, the attempt to discard the epidemiological population study, which remains crucial to the argument supporting mass vaccination, in favor of the clinical case study begins to look like a reaction to an increasingly bureaucratized medical and public health system. These activists have lost their trust in many health professionals because at their individual level, the policies do not work; knowing that your situation is statistically rare does not help. In this, they share in the long tradition of anti-vaccinationism in the United States: the individual patient (or vaccine recipient) must be valued more highly than the abstract population.[2]

The goals, then, of Dissatisfied Parents Together have remained relatively modest: to make vaccination safer and to help provide reliable legal recourse when, as they predict will happen, vaccinations turn out not to be so safe, after all. Their initial focus was on vaccine safety, and it remains their main goal. Short of eliminating the public health and legal requirements for pertussis vaccination, and making it entirely voluntary (as it is in Britain, for example), one of the consistent goals of Dissatisfied Parents Together has been to at least meliorate the effects of vaccine use. This has necessitated an engagement with the nature of vaccination, our cultural understanding of risk, and an attempt to change the way we respond to issues of vaccine safety.

Socially Constructing Challenges to Vaccine Safety

Americans' skepticism about vaccination safety has varied over time, depending on the particular disease, whether there is an ongoing epidemic (or a likely threat of one), political affiliation, attitudes about the appropriate role of government, religious beliefs, and the reputation of the health professions. Almost certainly, the zenith of popular enthusiasm for vaccines in the United States came on the heels of the Salk polio trials in the mid-1950s. Even during the Cutter incident, when hundreds of people contracted polio and several died from a bad batch of polio vaccine (Nathanson and Langmuir 1963), popular support hardly wavered—parents continued to line up their children to receive the vaccine. General support for vaccines has remained high since then, and while middle America has developed some qualms about vaccination, they do not seem nearly as concerned about efficacy as they do about safety, and vaccine compliance rates continue to be at historically high levels. Although vaccines remain one of the safest interventions with very small risks to the population as a whole, other aspects of public health and medicine have raised serious concerns about trust for health professionals. Vaccine opponents, whatever their objections, have almost always insisted that safety is a leading concern. These other issues have also helped change the calculus when it comes to vaccine safety.

The issue was never whether safety or efficacy is more important, but how the two relate, and how Americans value them. A cursory comparison between the United States and Britain reveals very different attitudes towards the interpretation of that relationship with regard to vaccines. In the twentieth century, the British have generally judged vaccine safety and efficacy to be equally important. British researchers and policymakers have evaluated vaccines in a calculus that compared the risk of adverse effects to the actual likelihood of contracting the disease based on its current prevalence, and the possibilities for effective treatment. In the U.S., following the pattern established in early smallpox vaccination and continuing through mass vaccination programs at the beginning of the twentieth century, safety has been secondary to, had a lower standard of proof than, and been almost entirely contingent on efficacy (Baker 2000). The American view has also emphasized the safety of each vaccine relative to a full-blown case of the disease, without taking into account the current risk of contracting it. For the British, then, as the risk of contracting pertussis declines, the calculus changes; American vaccine proponents have continued to compare the risks of adverse effect to a full-blown case of the disease when determining whether to continue pertussis vaccination policies (Barrie 1983; Fulginiti 1983; Marks 1997).

Attitudes towards medicine in general have passed through an arc of enthusiastic support that have, since the late 1960s, increasingly become skeptical about the ethical integrity of science and its practitioners. Publicity about birth defects associated with thalidomide in the late 1950s sparked public outrage and Congressional interest: otherwise healthy children were born with serious deformities (some were born without limbs) as a result of their mothers having been prescribed thalidomide to prevent morning sickness during pregnancy. In addition, there were statutory changes. The Kefauver hearings in the US Senate, as they came to be known for their chair Estes Kefauver, set out to investigate and reform safety protocols in the pharmaceutical industry. In 1962, in response to the thalidomide scandal, as well as to concerns about rising costs (and profits) associated with pharmaceuticals, Congress passed the "Kefauver-Harris amendments" to the 1938 Food, Drug, and Cosmetics Act. This provided new safety-testing guidelines for drugs and vaccines, including requirements for the clinical testing of all drugs to insure efficacy and safety (Asbury 1985). In this, for the first time, proof of safety began to approach the evidentiary status of efficacy in the United States: the law required statistical evidence of both. The highly publicized revelations about medical abuses of research subjects (Beecher 1966), including the Tuskegee Syphilis Study (Jones 1981) and the Willowbrook scandal (Rothman and Rothman 1984), together with growing grassroots movements to empower patients (e.g. Boston Women's Health Book Collective 1984) and changes in institutional frameworks (Rothman 1991), contributed to the weakening general faith in medical institutions and policies. Into this evolving context, parents of children vaccinated against pertussis who recognized adverse reactions began to take action about it.

Their public activism, though impressive compared to other recent attempts to oppose mandatory vaccination, did not make much of a dent in the public's behaviors associated with acceptance of vaccination. Reports, like "DPT: Vaccine Roulette," and a flow of new print and Internet publications questioning vaccine safety have sown some doubts about vaccination, but these strategies, by themselves, have had relatively little impact on the content of the cultural narrative. New vaccines continue to appear, with compliance rates staying at historically high levels. Alongside more direct publicity attempts, which have served important mobilization and consciousness-raising purposes, Dissatisfied Parents Together activists also used the courts as a way to gain publicity and to seek direct compensatory damages from vaccine manufacturers. The illness and death that followed vaccination with polio vaccine manufactured by Cutter Pharmaceuticals had established the legal precedent of "implied warranty" (Smith 1990). This holds that "if an injury is determined to be caused by the administration of a product—not necessarily on the basis of scientific proof—the producer is liable irrespective of the regulations, requirements, or level of testing performed before the product was entered into the market" (Murray 1969, 336). The exclusion of scientific proof as a requirement for judgment against a defendant meant not simply that a different standard of proof could be applied in the courts than in the laboratories, but that non-scientists (people who were not experts) were capable of making decisions about the validity of evidentiary claims relating to scientific cause and effect. Under these legal criteria, pertussis vaccine victims had ample standing to sue and possibly win large awards; there was an opening in the legal system that they had not found in the health professions. This strategy achieved more concrete successes than attempts to change vaccination policies directly.

Given the different threshold for proof in the courtroom, coupled with evidence from the peer reviewed literature and dramatic stories of children with life-long problems, legal actions against vaccine manufacturers began to win. Aside from individual awards, which might help compensate individual families, the cumulative effect of decisions based on adverse reactions to vaccines began to take their toll on the vaccine industry. In 1986, Dissatisfied Parents Together helped bring vaccine manufacturers and government officials to the negotiating table—not on technical or scientific issues, but on the issue of compensation for adverse reactions associated with childhood vaccines. The result, the National Childhood Vaccine Injury Act of 1986 (NCVIA) created a no-fault system for dealing with adverse reaction claims. Though it has been viewed as inadequate in many ways (e.g., Inglhart 1987), the NCVIA holds important symbolic meaning for vaccine opponents (Coulter and Fisher 1991; Fisher 2000). It recognized the incidence of adverse reactions—at least in the legal realm—though without assigning blame. A compromise, the NCVIA also placated pharmaceutical companies that had been complaining about the tort claims against them; the NCVIA limited initial damages using a "no fault" system and helped make the costs associated with such claims more predictable. The NCVIA provided for a panel that included parents of children injured by vaccines, and this meant a continuing voice in the adjudication of claims (IOM 1985). According to the DPT/NVIC website, $1.5 billion has been awarded to more than 120 claimants under the system by 2004 (NVIC). But for Dissatisfied Parents Together, money was never the central issue.

Perhaps the most crucial provision of the NCVIA for activists was that it mandated an unbiased scientific investigation of claims that pertussis and other vaccines were responsible for hitherto unrecognized adverse effects. In this, Dissatisfied Parents Together got what they said they wanted—an objective evaluation of the safety of pertussis vaccine. The Institute of Medicine (IOM), an arm of the National Academy of Sciences, conducted a series of studies commissioned by the NCVIA, in an attempt to use "accepted science" to settle once and for all claims about the dangers of vaccination, with an authoritative voice (Howson, Howe, and Fineberg 1991; Stratton, Howe, and Johnston 1994a, 1994b, 1994c). When the authoritative analyses had been completed, however, the only vaccine for which adverse reactions were confirmed was rubella vaccine—which the IOM found causes acute and chronic arthritis—and that mention occurred in a small footnote (Stratton, Howe, and Johnston 1994a). Those studies did not, however, produce the results that activists had hoped for with regard to pertussis vaccine; they found no causal relationship between pertussis vaccine and severe neurological damage and death.

Despite the IOM findings, however, pertussis vaccine did change, in 1996. In keeping with the idea that they advocate not for the elimination of vaccines, but for safer vaccines, Dissatisfied Parents Together activists have consistently argued for a safer form for the vaccine in use in the United States, which had been essentially unchanged since the 1940s. An alternative version, already in use in other countries by the mid-1980s, was an acellular pertussis vaccine that had a better track record on adverse reactions. In 1996, the FDA licensed the use of this version of pertussis vaccine (known as the DTaP vaccine), and it has since replaced the older vaccine (the one with all the adverse peer reviewed research). For Dissatisfied Parents Together, this was a major victory—activism has forced a change in vaccination practices on the basis of safety.

Opposition's Effect on the Narrative

To read about Dissatisfied Parents Together and their attempts to influence pertussis vaccine policies, it might seem that the vaccine narrative is not so resilient after all—it takes little more than a small group of dedicated people with a compelling counter-narrative to create crisis and even accomplish important changes in the ways that vaccines work in American society. So far, however, the changes have been largely about the implementation of vaccine use, rather than any fundamental challenge to vaccination in all its forms, as earlier anti-vaccinationists had advocated (Colgrove 2006). Compliance with mandatory and even voluntary vaccination remains high, and there is little evidence that faith in the narrative of vaccines—that is, the beneficent outcome of the story of vaccines—has changed. Dissatisfied Parents Together continues to propose an alternative to the master narrative, despite the changes in compensation law and improvements in the safety of pertussis vaccine itself: for them, the story of vaccination does not end with a healthy, disease-free society. Instead, Dissatisfied Parents Together asserts an ending in which science remains dominant, but works to uncover the dangers of vaccination. They insist that there needs to be a broader call for

> government funding of independent researchers to investigate the reported links between vaccines and neurological and autoimmune disorders, including learning disabilities, attention deficit disorder, autism, asthma, diabetes, otitis media, multiple sclerosis, lupus, Crohn's disease (intestinal disorders), chronic fatigue syndrome, rheumatoid arthritis, Alzheimer's, cancer, AIDS, Gulf War syndrome, personality disorders and other autoimmune and brain dysfunction which has been associated with vaccination. (NVIC)

This laundry list of adverse effects suggests a continuing and serious distrust of vaccines and their effects—a very different ending to the vaccine narrative, indeed.

The conflict between powerful and authoritative health institutions that support vaccination—and have supported it for more than a century—and the grass-roots movement that has opposed pertussis vaccination is about more than the individual members of the organizations and their desire to be free of public health regulations. It is a contest for the faith and trust of the American people—at least in terms of vaccines. At the nexus of both the pro- and anti-pertussis vaccination movements is the parent or guardian who must make decisions about whether or not to vaccinate. These average people can be influenced (as by the 1982 NBC television broadcast) to the benefit of a very small and otherwise powerless group, if the issue is perceived to be of general interest. Similarly, by using the court system to apply financial pressure on industry resources, activists were able to bargain with an otherwise implacable and unassailable group of institutions and authorities to some success (Burstein, Einwohner, and Hollander 1995). Thus, the anti-pertussis vaccine movement in the U.S. was able to engage with the widely accepted and powerful support for vaccines. The activism of Dissatisfied Parents Together compelled medical authorities to re-evaluate their fixed definition of "safety."

One of the almost incidental outcomes of the anti-pertussis vaccine movement since the formation of Dissatisfied Parents Together has been an increase in accessible information for parents (or anyone) interested in weighing the risks and benefits of vaccination in general, and this means that alternative views of vaccines are much more present in the culture. Numerous self-help-style books, each written from a slightly different perspective, address questions about *The Immunization Decision* (Neustaedter 1990) and promise to provide *What Every Parent Should Know About Childhood Immunization* (Murphy 1993)—even as scores of mainstream publications that fill the shelves of medical schools and physicians' offices continue to insist unequivocally on complete coverage with all approved vaccinations (e.g., Oski 1990; AAP 1994; Hoeckelman 1997).

Science-based opposition to pertussis vaccine, made possible in part by the documentation of existing scientific research questioning its safety, was the "breakthrough" event that has facilitated similar opposition to other vaccines. From the base established in Dissatisfied Parents Together, the National Vaccine Information Center has broadened the scope of its own mandate to encompass all mandatory vaccinations. This movement suggests the extent to which the rhetoric and language of science can be important for the success of a position that had, to all intents and purposes, been sent to the dustbin of history on the basis of scientific research, consensus among experts and policymakers, and a widespread faith that each new (or old) vaccine leads to better health for the individual and the general population. The standard argument defending pertussis vaccine has always been that because "no drug is totally safe, a risk exists with each dose of vaccine" (Altman 1982). This construction of the issue attempts, ironically, to remove the locus of contention away from the actual scientific evidence (where vaccine critics wanted to joust) and toward the far less objective grounds on which risks can be debated.

Dissatisfied Parents Together is proud of its achievements in terms of enactment of the NCVIA, the widespread use of the safer acellular pertussis vaccine, and cultural consciousness raising about the hazards of vaccination. These achievements are, indeed, impressive, especially considering the size of their organization and the authority and reach of the institutions supporting vaccination. More interesting for an under-standing of our cultural attitudes about the provenance of vaccines is that as a result of the concerted, science-based offensive, pertussis vac-cine *advocates* made changes in their strategies for promoting vaccine use. Vaccine proponents emerged from the privileged space in which scientific experts control the consensus and where science is the govern-ing factor to respond to the concerted challenge that seemed to show potential for destabilizing public perceptions of vaccines as safe, desir-able, and necessary.

The course of events surrounding modern contention around per-tussis vaccine also highlights the ways in which the health professions responded to challenges to vaccine safety. The public conflict over use of pertussis vaccine revealed vaccine proponents that were reluctant to revise their own conclusions about safety. Though scientific con-cerns continue to play an important part in the continuing discourse about vaccines, Americans' cultural judgments about their value (in the legal courts, and in the "court of public opinion") can easily be at variance with expert evaluations. Despite professional awareness of the risks associated with pertussis vaccine, those risks remained un-disclosed for fear that explaining the whole truth of pertussis vaccine, including the known risks, would undermine faith in vaccines gener-ally. Perhaps the ability to rationalize less-than-full disclosure about the probability of brain damage as one possible consequence of per-tussis vaccine, however small, was highly rational; that is: the benefits made it worth the risks. As the contention around pertussis vaccine played itself out, it became clear that at least part of the response to anti-pertussis vaccine activism was in defense not of the vaccine itself, but of the strong cultural narrative that insists that vaccines are effective, and therefore *always* worth it.

Other groups have expanded upon the kind of oppositional movement that anti-pertussis vaccine activists initiated in the early 1980s, and have taken it to higher levels, most notably as part of the lay movement to influence AIDS research. Beginning in the late 1980s, AIDS activists made impressive inroads among scientific experts, ultimately working as partners with researchers in the medical and research decision-making process. Their oppositional activity, which at some points centered on the development of a preventive HIV/AIDS vaccine (see Chapter 4), took a wide variety of forms, from confrontation to cooperation with health professionals, researchers, and policymakers[3] (Epstein 1996). AIDS activists, though using strategies and attitudes towards science similar to those used by Dissatisfied Parents Together, certainly did not challenge the vaccine narrative. In fact, most AIDS activists embraced the vaccine narrative in its entirety, ultimately demanding a vaccine as a right, perhaps hoping that once the vaccine narrative had been triggered, it would proceed to an inevitable conclusion: the eradication of AIDS.

4

HIV/AIDS Vaccine Research
Science and Ethics Confront the Narrative

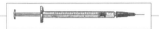

But the best hope the world has to thwart [HIV] is the same weapon effectively used against smallpox, polio, hepatitis B, rabies and other devastating viruses: a vaccine.

—Jon Cohen (2001)

▮ HIV/AIDS: A New Iteration of an Old Story

Americans came out of the 1960s and 1970s with a new complacence about their relationship to disease. Between antibiotics for bacterial infections and vaccines to protect against viruses, people supposed with good reason that dangerous infectious disease had been relegated to the history books (Sontag 1989). Smallpox's eradication in 1977 anticipated the same fate for other diseases; even the ongoing epidemics of venereal disease (syphilis and gonorrhea) were curable on a case-by-case basis with a simple course of antibiotics. Chronic, environmental, non-communicable, and lifestyle-related conditions, like heart disease and cancers, continued to confront society. But the evidence appeared clear that modern medicine had delivered the goods as promised: a population protected from random disease, as healthy as it was willing to be. At the same time, medical researchers and medicine in general had begun a slow but marked decline in prestige and influence (Rothman 1991; Schlesinger 2002). In a world without dangerous epidemics and in which the major public health measures included convincing people to wear seatbelts, get regular exercise, and eat vegetables, it is perhaps not surprising to find waning status for health professionals.

Then, in June of 1981, the Centers for Disease Control (CDC) quietly reported what looked like a deadly new communicable disease among homosexual men (CDC 1981). Soon it came to be known as AIDS (Acquired Immune Deficiency Syndrome), and a consensus emerged that it was caused by a retrovirus called HIV (Human Immunodeficiency Virus) and could be transmitted by sexual contact or through contact with infected blood. Early on, researchers discovered that HIV/AIDS disabled the immune system, it was nearly one hundred percent fatal, and the virus that caused it mutated quickly and often (Marx 1985).[1] With fear and hopeful expectation, Americans turned to the same medical profession that had defeated previous infectious diseases for a cure, an explanation, and protection. Some sectors of society reacted to AIDS more slowly than others. The earliest pleas for help with the new epidemic came from a small handful of researchers and from within the afflicted population. They found a medical research complex largely uninterested in applying its expertise and resources to the problem (Shilts 1987).

Within the United States, the status of people with HIV/AIDS was crucial for the nature of the response. Unlike polio, which were so closely associated with children, or smallpox and tuberculosis, which could be caught by casual contact, HIV/AIDS was quickly discovered to be difficult to transmit, so many people with AIDS found themselves labeled "responsible" for having contracted the disease. (Leary and Schreindorfer 1998). Biologically unlike any other human disease, HIV/AIDS had a close analog in terms of its social meaning: syphilis (Brandt 1988a, 1988b). Both HIV/AIDS and syphilis struck (or were at any rate generally perceived to strike) already marginalized groups and were transmitted primarily by particular behaviors (blood and sexual contact). Because of the way they spread, both diseases also divided the disease victims into "guilty" and "innocent" categories. For syphilis, this meant that preventive measures were politically difficult to formulate, let alone implement (Brandt 1985), and similar problems might be anticipated for HIV/AIDS.[2]

Ideas about how to contend with HIV/AIDS and its epidemic implications came quickly, but broke according to the perception of the problem. The clearest separation was between the communities suffering with AIDS and the general population potentially threatened by HIV, which for many years remained uninterested. Throughout the 1980s, for most Americans, HIV/AIDS remained bracketed off as a disease of gay men and drug users who had engaged in irresponsible behavior, or a disease of innocent victims (like hemophiliacs), who had contracted the disease through circumstances beyond their control (Palca 1992d). For some, like conservative commentator William F. Buckley, Jr., the problem was simple: stop the spread of the disease. In 1986, Buckley suggested that the government engrave a suitable tattoo on the forearm or on the buttocks of every drug user and every gay man infected with HIV (Buckley 1986). This idea, criticized at the time as "an astonishingly nasty bit of demagoguery" (NYT 1986), captured and unintentionally caricatured at least part of the general public's attitude towards HIV/AIDS: stop the people (drug addicts and gay men) from spreading it without worrying about the people who already have the disease. Those already infected found themselves stigmatized with a moral judgment on top of the disease itself; they also found themselves relatively alone in their concerns about HIV/AIDS as a public health problem. Together with a small group of dedicated advocates, people with AIDS worked to achieve recognition for the disease and its victims as well as to obtain resources for palliatives, treatments, cures, and preventives.

Because there were no effective drugs to treat, cure, or prevent HIV/AIDS, immediate responses to HIV/AIDS focused on education—knowledge as power—both for preventing the spread of the disease and for increasing tolerance and understanding of people with AIDS. Education would reduce panic, bring high-quality information to those who needed it most (people both infected and at risk) and help bring society together in an effort to halt the epidemic and cure the afflicted. Education aimed at preventing the transmission of HIV meant frank discussion of sexual behaviors, easy access to contraception, free needle exchanges for injection-drug users, and acknowledgement of alternative sexual lifestyles (Petit 1986; IOM 1986; Holden 1995). In the political and social climate of the 1980s, these kinds of strategies were, outside enclaves within places like San Francisco, New York, and Los Angeles, impractical, to say the least.

There was a simpler and longer-term solution, and one that everyone could agree upon. Medical science had contended with deadly contagious epidemics before; why couldn't the same model be used for HIV/AIDS? Since the 1920s, it had turned out to be cheaper and socially less disruptive to vaccinate a population living in squalor than to upgrade their living conditions, improve their educational institutions, or remove health hazards from the workplace. The same calculus applied in the 1980s. By the late twentieth century, alternatives like quarantine, stamping out, broader changes in social policies, or behavioral changes had all given way to one relatively inexpensive intervention against infectious disease: vaccination. Despite the erosion of popular trust in medicine, the public—and certainly medical and public health institutions—retained their faith in vaccines (Shorter 1987; Smith, Chu, and Barker 2004).

Moreover, the vaccine response contained all the elements to return to Americans their sense of invulnerability to infectious disease. A preventive HIV/AIDS vaccine promised an effective, safe, and painless way to rid the entire population of HIV/AIDS; it appealed to the broad spectrum of groups concerned about the disease and its social ramifications. There need be no inquiries into private sexual practices, no stigmatized categories of "guilty" and "innocent" victims: all would be protected equally and democratically. Vaccination obviated mentioning anal sex to junior-high-school and middle-school students or distributing hypodermic needles in communities wracked by injection-drug use. A vaccine also promised swift eradication of a deadly disease, which was the main point. A vaccine response to HIV/AIDS appeared to be a solution to the thorny social, political, public health, and medical issues. Because infection with HIV seemed inexorably to lead to AIDS, which was fatal, the idea of a vaccine preventive became still more attractive: a very powerful ounce of prevention. Americans knew how the HIV/AIDS vaccine story would progress: researchers would dedicate themselves to finding—and by dint of their efforts, would develop—a vaccine. The vaccine would be effective, safe, and provide lifelong immunity. Compliance with mass vaccination programs would dispatch AIDS just as previous vaccination campaigns had done with other infectious diseases; it could erase the whole idea of AIDS as if it had never been. AIDS could become just another chapter in the vaccine narrative.

It is therefore no surprise that from the earliest days of the epidemic, scientific researchers, physicians, public health officials, and HIV/AIDS activists consistently held the idea of a preventive vaccine at the top of their priorities (e.g., Marx 1983; Cohen 1993c), even if vaccines did not always receive funding commensurate with hopes.[3] Because HIV/AIDS presented a difficult range of technical problems, few expected a vaccine to come quickly or easily, but they expected one nevertheless. There were steps to follow and hurdles to overcome. But, for both the research community and the general population the consensus was clear: "the development of an effective vaccine that can be administered to the whole population is the only hope of effectively controlling the spread of [HIV] infection" (Krim 1985, 5). Confidence was so high that some suggested a vaccine might by its effectiveness help resolve the controversies about the cause of AIDS (Marx 1984).

The search for an HIV/AIDS vaccine is particularly fascinating because both policymakers and researchers pursued a vaccine despite technical, social, ethical, and even methodological contraindications. In the professional literature, hopes, goals, and attitudes thoroughly espoused the vaccine narrative, and vaccine research followed a path that was faithful to it: researchers sincerely believed that a vaccine should, could, and would be the solution to deliver complete control of HIV/AIDS. Moreover, the continued pursuit of a vaccine had to contend with the fact that there were alternative preventives with established efficacy.[4]

▉ Confronting a New Disease

HIV/AIDS researchers made surprisingly fast progress on all fronts, especially considering the scarcity of resources. Less than two years elapsed between the CDC's 1981 report of the disease in American medical circles and reports that France's Pasteur Institute and the National Cancer Institute had isolated its putative cause: a retrovirus ultimately called Human Immunodeficiency Virus, or HIV (Barré-Sinoussi, Chermann, et al. 1983; Gallo, Salahuddin, et al. 1984; Marx 1984; Marx 1986). In an April 1984 public announcement of the discovery of the virus, Margaret Heckler, the Secretary of Health and Human Services, predicted that a vaccine would be available within two years. At that time the mechanisms connecting HIV and AIDS remained unknown and funding for all aspects of AIDS research remained low; vaccine research faced the same tight funding constraints as other areas of AIDS research. Heckler's public announcement dismayed many HIV/AIDS researchers, not because they disputed the goal of a vaccine, but because it raised expectations too high; they felt the time-frame of her prediction was premature and unrealistic (Norman 1985a).

Heckler's announcement served the purposes of political expedience for the Reagan administration by projecting a public image of effectiveness and hope: an image that relied on the promise of a vaccine. Predictions for a cure might bear the politically untenable burden of curing "guilty" homosexuals and injection-drug users. The vaccine option avoided public discussion of the lifestyles and practices that were associated with HIV/AIDS; it skirted the issues associated with public support for groups or behaviors that were politically untenable.[5] Heckler and Reagan doubtless believed that a vaccine would solve the HIV/AIDS crisis; the decision to announce a forthcoming vaccine was based in uncritical acceptance of the vaccine narrative even as it served political purposes. It also applied the narrative to HIV/AIDS. The public promise of a preventive vaccine re-cast HIV/AIDS as an old-fashioned, "simple" disease, by virtue of its placement within the narrative of vaccination: HIV/AIDS would be solved by disinterested science in the laboratory, not by activists.

With a vaccine as the officially sanctioned solution—the government response—HIV/AIDS fell neatly into its place in the vaccine master narrative. Because of the cultural association with childhood diseases and the recent eradication of smallpox, a vaccine conjured an image of innocents protected from a random and predatory disease, like children protected from polio. In fact, the cases through which vaccination had become Americans' prototypical answer to infectious diseases (e.g.

smallpox, diphtheria, polio) were all highly transmissible by casual contact. By contrast, HIV/AIDS was known quite early to spread only by intimate contact: sex or bodily fluids (Zagury, Bernard, and Leibowitch 1984). Heckler's promise for a vaccine would solve the HIV/AIDS crisis without reference to sexual orientation, drug use, race, gender, social stigma, or personal behavior. It reassured people with promises of quick action, but the nature of that action—a vaccine—also made AIDS seem manageable.

Within months of Heckler's announcement, drug and biotechnology companies began competing for access to the U.S. government's supply of HIV for use in vaccine studies. Activists wanted still more aggressive vaccine action and almost immediately criticized the U.S. government's licensing requirements (prerequisites to beginning research on both a blood test and a vaccine) as too strict and therefore hindering vaccine development (Culliton 1984). By early 1985, as an antibody test for HIV became available for use, reports described the U.S. Public Health Service as "working feverishly to develop a vaccine" (Holden 1985, 1182). Heckler's unrealistic and scientifically unwarranted promise for a vaccine had helped spur a *bona fide* research surge for a vaccine. Already, the main players in the vaccine effort were in place: government funding sources, researchers and regulators, private companies vying for resources in a race to develop a vaccine, and activists advocating for their own view of the best way to proceed against the disease (Epstein 1996). All were committed to and supportive of a vaccine solution to HIV/AIDS. The health professions literature echoed the general cultural enthusiasm for a vaccine.

Congress soon publicly placed "a high priority on vaccine development" and accordingly raised research funding levels (Norman 1986), even though scientists were quite certain, and had been certain since shortly after the virus had been identified, that realistic expectations placed the target date for an effective vaccine "ready for general use" back as far as the year 2000 (Norman 1985d, 1357). These pessimistic predictions had their basis in technical problems, not skepticism about the goal. Vaccines remained "one of the most competitive areas in AIDS research" (Barnes 1986a, 282), as "the public is eager for an AIDS vaccine and scientists are working furiously to produce one" (Barnes 1986c, 1149). Despite little or no data supporting the effectiveness of perinatal vaccines (that would prevent transmission from mothers to children) such trials were "broadly endorsed by AIDS researchers and activist groups alike—and . . . received strong support from Congress" (Cohen 1992d, 1568). By the late 1980s the prevailing pro-vaccine take on HIV/AIDS prevention drew the attention and support of one of the luminaries in the pantheon of vaccine pioneers. Polio vaccine hero Jonas Salk, actively engaged in one branch of HIV/AIDS vaccine research, declared in 1993 that a "prophylactic vaccine against human immunodeficiency virus (HIV) infection represents the best hope for controlling the continuing and devastating worldwide AIDS epidemic" (Salk, Bretscher, et al. 1993, 1270). These attitudes pervaded the literature. By the mid-1990s the global nature of the epidemic had begun to receive wider publicity and, "the development of a safe and effective AIDS vaccine [had] become an urgent international public health priority" (Koff 1994, 1335).

Enthusiasm for a vaccine could not by itself translate into an easily produced or tested vaccine, however. Along with exhortations about the importance and value of an HIV/AIDS vaccine came the periodic reminders that "the process toward developing a vaccine faces unusually difficult challenges in both technical and social realms" (Barnes 1986c, 1149). One of the most frustrating technical difficulties was the absence of a suitable animal model for testing any new vaccine preparations. According to established practices, before any human testing can begin, efficacy-by-analogy needs to be demonstrated. Since the early twentieth century, statistical and laboratory evidence of efficacy in animal models has been entrenched as the "gold standard" to establish vaccines and other drugs for subsequent human testing in clinical trials (Palca 1990). Using animals as surrogates, researchers try to approximate the effects of drugs and gauge toxicity levels prior to any experimentation on any human subjects.

HIV, however, turned out to be highly species-specific, and researchers remained unable to find any suitable animal surrogate that could be meaningfully infected with it. In 1984, researchers discovered that chimpanzees—an endangered species—could be infected with HIV (Alter, Eichberg, et al. 1984), though they do not develop AIDS, at least not for nearly a decade, nor reliably so (Kaiser 1995; Lee 1997). Researchers tried other animal models: marmosets (Gallo, Sarin et al. 1983), mice (Leonard, Abramczuk, et al. 1988; Mosier, Gulizia, et al. 1991), pigtail macaques (Barnes 1988, 721; Palca 1992b), cats (Cohen 1993f), and baboons (Barnett, Murthy, et al. 1994), among others (Merz 1987). Scientists even studied a related retrovirus, SIV (Simian Immunodeficiency Virus), in primates (Daniel, Letvin, et al. 1984). No surrogate-animal test or situation satisfied researchers, and this left a procedural void in the initial steps toward preventive vaccine.

Because HIV infection in humans usually resulted in death, the inherent dangers of using traditional vaccine preparations, usually made from killed or attenuated pathogens (bacteria or viruses), were drastically increased with HIV. As a consequence, vaccine researchers focused their energies almost entirely on a new kind of vaccine—a "subunit" vaccine (Barnes 1986c, 282). Such genetically engineered recombinant vaccines contain only part of the HIV protein coat (Lasky, Groopman, et al. 1986; Putney, Matthews, et al. 1986). Recent discoveries in recombinant DNA research enabled the manufacture of sophisticated subunit vaccine preparations, rather than the relatively crude killed vaccines that had been used with polio, measles, and hepatitis B. But even sophisticated genetic engineering did not guarantee success (Marx 1987); as *Science* reported in 1988 about preclinical testing of vaccine preparations made from HIV proteins, "it is not working for AIDS, at least not so far" (Barnes 1988, 719). The difficulty posed by the absence of a suitable animal model fed into social problems that tested the strength of ethical rules with ramifications beyond the laboratory.

The Ethical Challenge

The dynamic equilibrium between method and ethics necessitates compromise in both areas, but over the years the balance has increasingly favored ethical concerns and strictly limited the ability of researchers to conduct what might otherwise be much more efficient and definitive studies. By the advent of HIV/AIDS, researchers had moved beyond the traditions of the "lesser harms" standard prevalent through the middle of the twentieth century (Halpern 2005), and mature and specific ethical codes of conduct governed their actions when contending with the new disease. Consequently, when HIV/AIDS vaccine research began in earnest, researchers had to contend with a more complex and restrictive set of ethical constraints than in any previous vaccine research campaign.

These ethical constraints stemmed less from abstract ideas about right and wrong than from the recent history of abuse in human-subjects research. In the 1960s, Senate hearings into deaths and birth defects caused by thalidomide (a drug designed to prevent miscarriage) resulted in changes to the 1938 Food, Drug, and Cosmetics Act to require testing to insure safety, as well as efficacy (Times of London 1979; Asbury 1985). Revelations about ethical abuses ranged from muckraking physicians to journalistic exposés (Beecher 1966; Jones 1981). Perhaps the most egregious example of abuse of informed consent rules happened during vaccine studies conducted at the Willowbrook State School for the Retarded, in which researchers intentionally infected children with hepatitis (Rothman and Rothman 1984). Most importantly for HIV/ AIDS vaccine research, sensitivity to the issues of informed consent and patient safety made the continued use of vulnerable populations within the United States politically and practically much more difficult. Certainly by the late 1970s, the flattering view of the medical researcher as hero had begun to come apart. The series of revelations about patient abuses resulted in clear and strong protections for human subjects under four main principles: informed consent, beneficence/non-maleficence, privacy, and justice (Campbell 1975; Annas and Grodin 1992; Beauchamp and Childress 1994; Macklin 2004). (See Table 1.)

The ethical principle that first caused contention in HIV/AIDS vaccine research was a subsidiary class of the beneficence and non-maleficence principles, called *equipoise*, because it had direct implications for research methodologies. The equipoise standard requires that control subjects receive better than the equivalent of sugar-pill placebos. Instead, they must be given the best alternative therapy or preventive; anything less would amount to denying research subjects treatment or access to preventive measures, and therefore harming them (Hutchins and Eckes 1994). In light of this standard, the IOM (Institute of Medicine, the research arm of the National Academy of

Table 1	Ethical Principles Briefly Described (NCPHSBBR 1978)
Informed Consent	Each individual (or a duly authorized representative of that person's interest; for example, a parent may consent for a child) must be treated as an autonomous agent, supplied with all necessary information about purposes, risks, incentives, and likely outcomes of the particular research plan to guarantee voluntary participation; persons with diminished autonomy are entitled to protection.
Beneficence/ Non-Maleficence	Research efforts must promise to protect and promote subjects' well being, as well as to "do no harm." Under the sub-heading of equipoise, no subject may be denied access to treatments or preventives as a consequence of participation in research studies.
Privacy	Research subjects must be guaranteed both privacy and confidentiality. Researchers have no right to access information about subjects' behaviors, practices, or beliefs without explicit consent under the informed consent requirement. Any private information that subjects do reveal must be kept in complete confidence.
Justice	Research subjects must be selected equitably without bias, and must potentially share in the fruits of research.

Sciences) directed that education and counseling qualified as an effective preventive to HIV infection. The IOM declared that "ethical considerations also dictate that those who receive the vaccine must be counseled about behavior changes that diminish the chance for HIV infection" (IOM 1988a, 145). Because of the necessity for any vaccine clinical field trials to be double-blind, researchers would have to counsel all subjects, both test and control, about ways to reduce the chance of HIV infection through behavioral changes, appropriate to the local epidemiology. Such action affected one of the most important scientific factors that made test populations attractive for vaccine trials: it threatened to reduce infection rates.

High infection rates were desirable because without them, clinical trials of a vaccine candidate would become unworkable. Despite technological advances and improved understanding of how vaccines work, the basic principle underlying human vaccine trials had hardly changed since the first decades of the twentieth century; randomized, controlled clinical trials were the necessary proving ground after laboratory experiments had determined vaccine efficacy. After suitable animal testing to establish measurable levels of vaccine efficacy, a vaccine candidate must pass three phases of human testing before it may be considered for general use. Phase I clinical vaccine trials test for toxicity (safety), and are carried out on small numbers of volunteers under close laboratory supervision. Phase II trials are carried out on a larger volunteer population to determine proper dosages as well as timing between doses, though still within a laboratory-based setting. Phase III trials are clinical field trials, carried out on large numbers of people in an active population, to test for vaccine efficacy: Does the vaccine confer measurable and sufficient protection in controlled real-world situations? Successful Phase III trials are crucial to moving a vaccine from the experimental stage into production and general use (Putney and Bolognesi 1990). It is during Phase III trials, then, that infection rates become important.

Planning Human Vaccine Trials— Altering Established Standards

Anticipation of Phase III vaccine trials in the United States meant that large numbers of volunteers, necessarily including people at high risk for HIV infection, would be required (Koff and Hoth 1988). The logical source for trial participants would therefore come from the gay and injection-drug-using populations in the United States and Europe, or the hard-hit areas in Africa. Two immediate and interconnected problems emerged. The first problem had to do with compliance with ethical standards. The IOM rules guaranteeing equipoise meant that all vaccine trial subjects would have to receive behavioral counseling about how to reduce the chances of contracting HIV. Education and behavioral counseling might slow or interrupt transmission of HIV/AIDS; the ethical requirements of equipoise would force vaccine researchers to provide such "behavioral protection" to both test and control populations. This would be a good thing for the research subjects, and a highly ethical practice, but it presented a seemingly insurmountable impediment to vaccine research. Randomized clinical vaccine trials ask researchers to compare experimental and control groups in an active population that are as similar as possible in all measurable attributes except for the test variable (in this case, an HIV/AIDS vaccine candidate); this is the essence of the scientific method (Goldstein and Goldstein 1980). Ideally, such field trials would be under double-blind conditions in which the experimental group receives an HIV/AIDS vaccine candidate, and the control group receives a placebo (Koff and Hoth 1988). The method is simple and capable of producing reliable results. Reduced risks of infection, however, would make rigorous studies leading to a preventive HIV/AIDS vaccine increasingly difficult or impossible. Clinical vaccine trials rely on a measurable level of infection in the test population, without which there is no basis for comparison, and no gauge for the effectiveness of the vaccine candidate.

In fact, counseling about safe-sex practices, including condom use, worked quite well in some communities at stopping the spread of HIV/AIDS (Judson 1983; CDC 1984; Curran, Morgan, et al. 1985). This presented the second problem: by the time that researchers began to think they had viable vaccine candidates, the accessible American populations had already reduced their transmission rates. Education efforts had not reached all Americans equally, however, and unlike the gay community, racial and ethnic minorities had not benefited from HIV/AIDS education efforts. These groups remained skeptical about accepting advice from mainstream researchers, at least in part because of the long history of being exploited in medical research (Stolberg 1998). The charge that researchers were racist in the use of minority populations was not new to HIV/AIDS research (Thomas and Quinn 1987; Gamble 1991; Jones 1992; Benedek and Erlen 1999), but the abiding lack of trust that caused education and outreach interventions like needle-exchange programs to fail were also likely to cause similar problems in any vaccine-based initiative (Watters 1996). Though arguably the most suitable American test population in terms of infection rates, these subpopulations were generally unwilling to serve as "guinea pigs" for vaccine tests, and consequently difficult for vaccine researchers to use in field trials.

The unusual combination of a well-informed and highly motivated at-risk population with declining infection rates (the gay community), an inaccessible population with high infection rates (racial minorities), and an ethical standard that required researchers to inform subjects about behaviors that were effective at preventing the spread of disease made finding American research subjects for clinical vaccine trials almost impossible. As these researchers noted in 1988, the decreased incidence of infection among gay men meant lost opportunities to test a vaccine:

> If an AIDS vaccine had been available for testing in the United States 2 to 3 years ago in phase 3 clinical trials, the preferential population for testing might have been homosexual men at high risk for HIV infection; however, the incidence of infection in this population (because of education efforts) has now decreased. (Koff and Hoth 1988, 431)

Five years later, studies began to suggest that no vaccine could ever reach the levels of effectiveness achieved by the appropriate use of condoms (Pinkerton and Abramson 1993; Blower and McLean 1994). The effectiveness of behavior modification revived a method for containing the epidemic that did not rely on laboratories; it did not even need positive identification of the AIDS germ in order to work. Such technologically primitive measures posed a surprisingly strong challenge to vaccination. The existence of effective behavioral preventive measures, together with an enforced equipoise standard that would bring such measures to any research population, meant that rigorous, ethical vaccine trials would be difficult, if not impossible to stage.

Even as researchers encountered ethical and research protocol difficulties, AIDS activists were pressing for more research money, more research, and more results. In addition to reducing their transmission rates, gay men at risk for HIV in the United States also began to assert both their rights and availability as research subjects, thereby "changing the way that drugs move through the scientific and regulatory pipeline" (Booth 1988b, 1279). Though a research subject's ability to make an informed decision about participation in research is one of the cornerstones of biomedical ethics (see Table 1), too much participation threatens the authority of the researcher, and can undermine the methodological rigor of clinical trials. The activism and knowledge about the disease possessed by many Americans at risk for HIV/AIDS made them less than suitable as research subjects; they were much more difficult to deal with (Volberding and Abrams 1985). Despite pleas from spokespeople like Larry Kramer to "let us be your guinea pigs" (Booth 1988a), many AIDS activists remained more focused on saving lives than following the particular protocols called for in scientific studies. Jim Eigo, one of the leaders of ACT UP (AIDS Coalition to Unleash Power), argued for the need to help people with AIDS, instead of being "in awe of the 'strange and abstract god, clean data'" (Marshall 1989, 345). It was "clean data," however, that researchers needed in order to develop a vaccine that worked.

According to the narrative, a vaccine was not supposed to take so long. Fairly quickly, the scientific establishment, including drug regulators, began to agree with Eigo's attitude. The long incubation period for AIDS (five or more years, in some cases) combined with expectations for a vaccine to impel federal drug-licensing agencies to reduce the established evidentiary thresholds for human vaccine trials. Existing standards required animal-experimentation evidence of efficacy before tests could be conducted on human subjects. For an HIV/AIDS vaccine, this would have required an extremely expensive, time-consuming "chimpanzee challenge," or other standard animal efficacy tests, to establish protective efficacy (IOM 1986). In such an experiment, vaccinated test animals would be challenged with live HIV to determine whether the vaccine conferred immunity to infection (Palca 1992a). With a lag time between infection and the development of symptoms of up to a decade, adhering to these standards of proof would push a vaccine into the distant future. To overcome this obstacle, HIV/AIDS vaccine candidates were permitted to progress to the next stage—the first phase of human experimentation in the proving process, Phase I trials—without passing the test of whether they prevented disease or infection.

This change in policies was not uncontroversial, and there was vocal dissent, including from luminaries like Albert Sabin, discoverer of the second polio vaccine (Sabin 1991), but the decision stood. A 1987 AIDS vaccine workshop sponsored by the U.S. Public Health Services and the U.S. Army Medical Research and Development Command focused on three questions that would be important in FDA (Food and Drug Administration) decisions certifying vaccines for use: 1) what is an acceptable endpoint for an AIDS vaccine trial? 2) how well do results of pre-clinical tests predict vaccine efficacy in humans? and 3) which human populations should receive test vaccines? (Barnes 1987b). The first question was technically the most difficult because it had to establish a new standard for efficacy. People infected with HIV or afflicted with AIDS initially produced prodigious antibody responses—the goal of any vaccine—"but they still get sick" (Haseltine in Barnes 1986c, 1152).

Infection with HIV seemed to lead inexorably to AIDS, and AIDS led just as inexorably to death. So in order to be effective, a vaccine would most likely need to prevent infection with HIV, not simply prevent progression to disease, as all previous vaccines had done. This level of protection was called sterilizing immunity. But there were serious technical difficulties with producing an HIV/AIDS vaccine, as well.

Some researchers made compelling arguments that, on the basis of technical problems, a preventive vaccine would never become a reality. The purpose of vaccination is to find a safer substance than the actual infecting germ to stimulate the production of antibodies against the disease, and therefore confer immunity. Jenner used cowpox to confer protection against smallpox, Park used a combination of diphtheria toxin and antitoxin, Salk used a killed polio virus. Because the AIDS virus was so lethal, fears of an insufficiently killed virus (as had happened in the Cutter accident during initial polio vaccination in 1955) made that option too dangerous to consider. The main alternative was to use only the "protein coat" from the AIDS virus. But because of the virus's rapid reproduction, and consequently frequent mutations, there were concerns that by using subunit vaccines that included only the protein coat from HIV, "a single vaccine might not be able to confer immunity to all strains" (Marx 1985, 1449). This meant that the virus's mutability could allow it to "elude protection offered by a vaccine" (Norman 1985a, 419). Moreover, most people suffering from AIDS already had high levels of antibodies in their blood (the basis for early AIDS blood tests), yet these antibodies did not appear to inhibit infection by the virus, and antibodies developed against one strain of HIV had no effect on other strains (Norman 1985e; Barnes 1986c). Unlike diseases like polio and smallpox, which were caused by stable germs, and for which surviving a case of the disease conferred lifelong immunity, HIV's mutability might make any vaccine only partially effective and only against some strains. Also, no one knew whether surviving a case of AIDS conferred immunity, because no one had survived a case of AIDS.

The technical problems of discovering an effective HIV/AIDS vaccine, therefore, were formidable. Nevertheless, the expectations for a vaccine ending to the HIV/AIDS story (i.e., the expectations of the vaccine narrative) made it possible for researchers to weaken their standards to achieve that end. Quickly, researchers began to use "surrogate endpoints," such as levels of particular kinds of cells involved in immunity to claim efficacy for vaccine candidates, rather than the ability to prevent disease (Cohen 1991b). The new, lower standards allowed human vaccine trials to proceed as far as Phase II. Rather than acknowledge the practical difficulties of developing an HIV/AIDS vaccine in the near future or the ethical quandary raised by the equipoise standards in a context with effective behavioral interventions, researchers and regulators reached a consensus to alter the ethical and methodological requirements for making a safe and effective vaccine.

Incentives for Vaccine Trials

A successful vaccine promised to be highly lucrative for the company that obtained the patent, and even the research process itself could be rewarding, as it attracted investors and provided status to researchers. Just two years after HIV had been identified, companies began their research programs. By 1986, Genentech, Inc. was already reporting preliminary findings about antibodies (Barnes 1986c), and a year later MicroGeneSys began Phase I testing of a vaccine candidate (Barnes 1987c). The realization that continued public funding for HIV/AIDS was, unlike for most other diseases, tied to some kind of demonstrated success with vaccines helped keep researchers focused on the goal despite the wide variety of factors that militated against it. Anthony Fauci, the director of NIAID (National Institute of Allergy and Infectious Diseases) and head of the new Office of AIDS Research at the NIH (National Institutes of Health) imagined research funding would "plateau sometime in 1992 or 1993 . . . unless a major breakthrough occurs in vaccine development" (Booth 1988c, 859). Perhaps this sentiment was felt more widely, because technical setbacks notwithstanding, vaccines remained at the forefront of research agendas, and "the pessimism shadowing the development of an AIDS vaccine [began] showing some signs of receding" (Bolognesi 1989, 246, 1233). By 1991, the greatest quantity of HIV being grown for research was for diagnostic testing and vaccine trials (Haseltine and Levy 1991). By 1992, positive reports of laboratory tests involving an old vaccine technique, an attenuated, whole-cell virus vaccine, reinvigorated the research establishment (Arthur, Bess, et al. 1992; Daniel, Kirchoff, et al. 1992; Cohen 1992g).

Companies eager to be the first to develop an effective vaccine awaited supplies of HIV challenge stock in order to proceed with their separate tests (Palca 1992a), and NIAID had begun putting into place the infrastructure necessary to conduct Phase III trials, when vaccine candidates reached that stage, though none were expected to be ready for such tests in the foreseeable future (Palca 1992c). Those doubts faded when Congress appropriated $20 million to study HIV/AIDS vaccines (Cohen 1992b). In the short term, the availability of funds changed the dynamics of vaccine research, and plans went ahead to test different vaccine candidates against one another, allowing inter-comparisons among them as well as compared to no vaccine (a placebo).

These trials would not test the newly promising attenuated vaccines, because they were nowhere near ready for Phase II trials. They would also not test vaccine candidates that might fulfill Heckler's (and the vaccine narrative's) promise of a preventive vaccine. Instead, the $20 million would fund trials of "therapeutic vaccine" candidates that three different companies, frustrated in their attempts to find a preventive vaccine, had begun to develop (Goldsmith 1991; Cohen 1992c). Not a vaccine in the common definition, a therapeutic vaccine would be a vaccine-like preparation, genetically engineered out of synthetic protein-coats to boost a person's immunity after infection had occurred.[6] One top NIH HIV/AIDS researcher admitted that if the new money "had not come along, [such trials] would not have been a high scientific priority to us." Researchers also expressed concern that the funding could affect the government's research progress and "skew its existing research program" away from finding a preventive vaccine (Cohen 1993b, 752). That was exactly what the money did. The move to begin testing of therapeutic vaccines marked a radical change in goals, though it maintained nominal adherence to the vaccine narrative: something called a vaccine might be produced. Moreover, the $20 million would be spent on trials for a therapeutic vaccine that had been held to only the new, lower standards of efficacy; they had no demonstrated ability to protect against the disease. NIH's own "blue ribbon panel concluded there [were] not enough hard data to justify a large-scale trial of a therapeutic AIDS vaccine. . . . But, after looking the gift horse in the mouth, the panel decided the money was too tempting to pass up," and voted to stage a multi-vaccine trial with the $20 million (Cohen 1992e).

With the $20 million on the table for therapeutic vaccine trials, NIH began in earnest to set up the necessary preparations for side-by-side trials of different subunit therapeutic vaccine candidates, produced by different companies and research labs. These sophisticated new preparations had been derived from HIV strains common in the United States, and in one case from a relatively rare American strain (Cohen 1992f).

Quickly, the planned trials ran into difficulties. Accusations of preferential treatment for one of the companies, MicroGeneSys, which did not want comparative trials (Stone 1993a), coupled with its attempt to sell supplies of vaccine to be used in the trials (Stone 1993c), roiled the political waters (vaccine stocks are typically donated for trials, not sold). After a turf struggle with the Department of Defense over the money, the NIH regained formal control of the trials and continued preparations for competitive trials (Cohen 1993d). At one point during contention over who should run the trials, the NIH admitted that "the fundamental reasons for doing the trial are on shaky ground" (Stone 1993b). Lay activists from ACT UP became involved and brought publicity to the planned trials, saying that one company, MicroGeneSys, had "bypassed the peer review process." This, together with testimony from NIH, led to legislation in Congress to reallocate the $20 million to different aspects of HIV/AIDS research altogether (Stone 1993d; Stone 1993e; Stone 1993f).

This outcome was a major reversal for companies hoping to have the government test and approve their vaccine candidates, but it was hailed as a triumph for the scientific rigor of the peer review process (Cohen 1993a). Government agencies had received unlooked-for support from AIDS activists. ACT UP had threatened "a massive boycott" of efficacy trials and charged that plans to go ahead with the trials were not only premature, but "extremely unethical and dangerous." Activists' opposition was based in part on fears that vaccines might enhance susceptibility to HIV, rather than confer benefits (Cohen 1994c), but it also reaffirmed their faith in the peer review process as the appropriate route for vaccines to follow. Scientific researchers, not companies or legislators, would make decisions about the development of vaccines.

The peer review process, however, continued to produce scientifically valid but disappointing results. At the 1993 annual AIDS vaccine conference in Alexandria, Virginia, vaccine developers received a serious setback as previously encouraging candidate vaccines failed to protect against field strains of HIV from actual people infected with HIV: they had shown some effectiveness against specific laboratory strains, but not against an approximation of what would be encountered in the real world (Cohen 1993f).

Companies Want Protection Too

The combination of disappointing laboratory results, NIH's decision to forego the $20 million, and NIAID's evaluation that there were no suitable candidates for vaccine trials made vaccine companies nervous. Vaccine manufacturers that had "scaled up operations" in anticipation of trials worried that these decisions could jeopardize their investments. The head of the AIDS project at Genentech, Inc., which had produced one of the vaccine candidates, argued that

To leave that vaccine on the shelf, something that might help some-one, we think that's ridiculous. . . . this is a monumental disincentive for Genentech. . . . What needs to be forthcoming is for NIH not to dawdle about, one step forward, one step back. That's what makes CEOs nervous. (Cohen 1993f)

These were not complaints about improper science or the failure of bureaucracies to respond to the needs of sick people. Leaving a vaccine candidate "on the shelf" cost companies money and credibility with investors, even if that vaccine showed little evidence of efficacy. De-spite sincere interest in producing a life-saving biologic, the profit mo-tive was crucial for companies involved in vaccine research: HIV/AIDS vaccine research had potentially high monetary rewards.[7] At the same time, companies feared losses. As one analyst of the ethics of HIV/AIDS research put it, the threat of tort liability was preventing "serious in-vestment in vaccine research" because vaccine manufacturers felt they needed to be "fiscally cautious" (Kerns 1997, 45). Exposure to tort li-ability was one of the most frequently mentioned concerns among com-panies pursuing vaccine research. The threat of lawsuits, according to the companies, imperiled their ability to conduct much needed research studies (e.g., IOM 1986; Barnes 1986a; Barnes 1987b; Stine 1993).

Liability concerns pre-dated the appearance of any viable vaccine candidates for HIV/AIDS. As early as 1986, at a time when HIV/AIDS funding was only gradually becoming more available and work was just beginning on a vaccine, issues of profit and costs for vaccine manufac-turer's had already become prominent. A *Science* magazine article titled "Will an AIDS Vaccine Bankrupt the Company that Makes It?" out-lined the view of vaccine manufacturers throughout the period: "In the present climate of richly rewarding lawsuits by individuals for product liability, US pharmaceutical companies may be less than eager to invest large amounts of money and effort into producing a vaccine for AIDS" (Barnes 1986b, 1035). The litigants in these "richly rewarding law-suits" had largely been claimants against pertussis vaccine manufactur-ers (IOM 1985; Sun 1986). The precedent under which they had made such claims against vaccine manufacturers went back to the 1950s. At that time, the courts had ruled that manufacturers could be held liable following adverse reactions to the Salk polio vaccine produced by Cut-ter Pharmaceuticals (Asbury 1985). Of course the polio precedent had neither limited subsequent polio vaccine development and use, nor the development of a broad range of other vaccines.

Potential HIV/AIDS vaccine manufacturers also pointed to their experience after the swine flu vaccine in 1976 as evidence of potential risks (Altman 1986; Kirp and Maher 1987; Shilts 1987). Their claim that the possibility of lawsuits posed a huge and immobilizing problem for vaccine manufacturers became the central non-scientific issue around vaccine research. This was especially the case when it came to testing vaccine candidates in Phase III trials, where exposure to tort liability would be multiplied by uncertainty about the effects of sub-unit retrovirus vaccines and the large number of trial participants. In response to these concerns and in an effort to foster research, California set up an AIDS Vaccine Victims Compensation Fund and even went so far as to pass a law limiting tort liability for AIDS vaccine manufacturers, under the assumption that such a vaccine would be "unavoidably dangerous" (Gostin 1989). HIV/AIDS vaccine researchers wanted these kinds of protections nationally.

The move to protect companies from liability opposed the long-standing right to sue for damages in American society—actions in tort. Assertions that "an AIDS vaccine never will be developed in this country unless its producers can be guaranteed immunity from or limits on liability for untoward results" (Gamble 1986, 31) pit the hope and promise of a preventive vaccine against the rights of research subjects to legal action as a form of recourse when they incurred injuries (adverse effects). A presidential commission on human subjects rights (separate from the HIV/AIDS context) reaffirmed the right to sue on grounds of both fairness and gratitude: "it would be 'morally preferable' not to insist that subjects waive the right to all claims of redress, particularly if no therapy is involved in the research" (PCSEPMBBR 1982, 3). Of course, there was no uncertainty about at least one aspect of the risks of participation in a Phase III clinical field trial: some measurable proportion of subjects would have to become infected with HIV (or, for a therapeutic vaccine trial, develop AIDS) if the trail was going to demonstrate whether the vaccine candidate worked. Subjects could not, of course, sue manufacturers for landing in the control group, but this was not the nature of the tort liability complaint. The lawsuits companies feared were from adverse effects of the vaccine itself.

Ethicists asserted a "right" to sue for compensation, arguing that "experimental subjects should never, in giving their consent to participation, be required to waive their rights to compensation in case of injury; nor should they be required to show negligence or lack of a reasonable degree of skill on the part of the investigator" (Dunne 1995, 218). But some members of Congress felt strongly enough that tort litigation was slowing development of a vaccine to introduce a bill "that would protect responsible manufacturers from costly lawsuits filed by recipients of experimental or approved vaccines," with plans to set up AIDS Vaccine Development and Compensation Program, based on the pertussis vaccine-inspired 1986 National Childhood Vaccine Injury Act (Cohen 1992e). Nevertheless, complaints about tort liability preventing development in an HIV/AIDS vaccine may well have been exaggerated.

Some evidence suggests that liability concerns were not keeping pharmaceutical companies out of the search for HIV/AIDS drugs and vaccines. A 1989 article in the *American Journal of Public Health* that was very supportive of the search for a vaccine (its desirability was "obvious"), noted that "the pace of HIV vaccine research is virtually unprecedented" and pointed out the irony that

> there have been more specific suggestions affecting the potential liability issue than the conduct of vaccine trials, in spite of the absence of evidence that liability poses a substantial obstacle to vaccine development. . . . in light of the number of researchers and producers studying approaches to AIDS vaccines and the number of years before a vaccine could become available, liability concerns seem tangential at present. (Mariner 1989, 90)

According to the Pharmaceutical Manufacturers Association, in 1989 nearly 60 companies had AIDS drugs or vaccines in development (Marx 1989).

Companies working on vaccine candidates nevertheless insisted that the imperative to create a vaccine superseded ethical concerns about compensation for injury. They needed protection from tort liability, and they were willing to consider foregoing trials in the United States to achieve their goal. Even as AIDS was "fast becoming the single largest program in the federal health bureaucracy" (Booth 1988c, 858)—that meant that American taxpayers were paying for lots of HIV/AIDS-related research—health professionals began discussing how

> the risks associated with vaccine trials have prompted some researchers to consider testing vaccines against HIV in countries of equatorial Africa, where the prevalence of infection is known to be higher than in the United States, and where the number of trial participants could therefore be lower. In addition, the risk of litigation for research-related injury might be reduced in a non-U.S. setting. However, the proposal to export research risks raises questions of fairness in its own right. (Walters 1988, 602)

The willingness to "export research" and its risks was not new in HIV/AIDS research. The idea that Phase III trials would be held in poorer and non-white areas of the world had taken hold early, based partly on the epidemiological logic—trials in a population at very high risk for infection can be faster, smaller, easier, and cheaper—but also based in a continuing public discussion that linked the dangers of litigation with the methodology of clinical vaccine trials. In 1992, at a vaccine development conference in Chantilly, Virginia, participants seriously questioned whether researchers would be able to recruit "the thousands of volunteers needed for large scale trials" from the American population of "homosexual men (especially those considered likely to practice unsafe sex) or intravenous drug users who share needles" (Palca 1992c, 1472). American politicians, researchers, and the American public all wanted an HIV/AIDS vaccine, as the inevitable conclusion promised by the familiar vaccine narrative. There was much less willingness to subject American subjects to the risks of that process, and drug companies were reluctant to take the financial risks of being sued by American subjects in order to test a vaccine. Instead, researchers would look outside the American population.

◼ The Search for Phase III Clinical Trial Subjects

With the realization that Phase III trials were going to be all but impossible in the United States because of scientific thresholds, ethical enforcement, and contributing liability concerns, it might seem that the vaccine effort had confronted immovable ethical and methodological obstacles. But the vaccine narrative does not end in defeat. Vaccine researchers therefore shifted their efforts to other populations where the research situation would be more conducive, and where they would have more autonomy. Unlike small-scale tests of preventive vaccines over the previous six years, which had "included only volunteers from low-risk groups" (Cohen 1992f), full field vaccine trials would require large numbers of people at high risk for infection. Vaccine manufacturers turned to WHO (the World Health Organization), which gave indications it might break with NIAID and lower its evidentiary thresholds of efficacy to allow Phase III vaccine trials, making it easier to proceed (Cohen 1993f).

Africa stood at the top of the list of potential sites for field trials—specifically Zaire, Rwanda, and Uganda, though Brazil and Thailand made the short list as well, and NIAID said it was "looking at the United States too" (Cohen 1991a, 647). Except for the United States, which had only specific and largely inaccessible subpopulations that shared the dubious distinction, these places shared an important common feature: high HIV infection rates.[8] High infection rates would amplify "the statistical power of the results and [provide] massive savings in time and money" (Nowak 1995, 1333). Researchers knew this and already had been very active; one survey estimated that by 1990, close to 600 different kinds of HIV/AIDS-related studies were underway in Africa (Palca 1990b). Because Africa had also received a great deal of attention as the probable origin of AIDS (Marx 1983; Brun-Vézinet, Rouzioux, et al. 1984; Norman 1985c) and was very hard hit by the epidemic, there appeared to be a kind of moral sense to seeking a vaccine there.

Devoting resources to HIV/AIDS research in Africa seemed to mean addressing the problem of HIV/AIDS in Africa. Indeed, a prodigious amount of research was certainly taking place in Africa, but it was not clear who benefited most from it. Under the ethical principle of justice, "research subjects should be chosen for reasons directly related to the problem being studied, and not because of their easy availability, their compromised position, or their manipulability" (Christakis 1988, 36). Yet these were precisely the reasons that researchers seemed interested in using populations in Africa, Thailand, and Brazil.

In response to concerns about the use of vulnerable subjects in HIV/AIDS research, in 1991 the U.S. Government promulgated a new Federal Policy for Protection of Human Subjects that required "any U.S. government-funded researcher at home or overseas [to] 'minimize the possibility of coercion or undue influence' of potential trial participants" (Nowak 1995, 1333). This imposed a kind of research ethics extraterritoriality. Unfortunately, even within the United States, standards like informed consent could be relatively weak: "as long as a patient does or says nothing strange and acquiesces to treatment recommended by the medical professional, questions of competency do not arise" (Drane 1985, 17). How they were understood and used abroad is a different story, because ethical rules do not translate easily across cultures.

The American conception of the informed consent principle, which requires researchers to provide sufficient information to each individual to make an autonomous decision about whether to participate in research program, does not export well—even to a cultural cousin like Britain (Schwartz and Grubb 1985), and apparently not at all to Japan (Feldman 1985). The American standards typically employed a stricter notion of the individual than those in general use. In eastern Africa, where HIV/AIDS had reached pandemic proportions, the idea of autonomous informed consent had to confront the problem even in semantic terms: "many Bantu languages lack terms corresponding to the English word 'person.' Personhood is defined by one's tribe, village, or social group" (Barry 1988, 1083). One Nigerian doctor recommended "uninformed consent," arguing that when a researcher cannot convince subjects "of the true etiology and pathology of the disease, he should not waste his time" (Ekunwe and Kessel 1984, 23). The practical difficulty of applying American ethical standards in the places in which HIV/AIDS vaccine trials were being planned presented a seemingly unavoidable obstacle to the ethical conduct of Phase III vaccine trials. It did not, however, mean that plans for such trials would not proceed.

In fact, Africa was the site of the first-ever HIV/AIDS vaccine trial, in 1987, conducted by Dr. Daniel Zagury, a French researcher with close ties to American researchers. Zagury administered a vaccine to a small group of Africans, apparently without any ethical oversight whatsoever.[9] The advantages for companies and researchers in selecting African sites were clear: ethical rules were easier to sidestep, final say about the selection of research subjects would be left to researchers without interference from institutional review boards or activists, and liability claims for injury were unlikely. Testing a vaccine in Africa, Brazil, or Thailand had many fewer constraints than testing the same vaccine in San Francisco.

Equipoise would not be addressed in vaccine trials outside the United States. Dr. Donald Francis, who had been active in HIV/AIDS research since the beginning of the epidemic (starting at the CDC), and who in the 1980s had argued eloquently for educational and behavioral methods of controlling the spread of HIV/AIDS in the United States (Francis and Chin 1987), came out against the equipoise standard when he worked for Genentech, Inc. in the 1990s: "We are testing the efficacy of a vaccine, we are not testing the efficacy of behavioral intervention." Francis argued that behavioral interventions should match the standards in the given community, "no more and no less" (Francis in Cohen 1994b, 1073). This would mean researchers withholding prevention information from African subjects because the subjects did not already generally have access to that information. Still, some voices kept alive the idea of comparable education and behavioral counseling programs for Africa (Quinn, Mann, et al. 1986; Culotta 1991). When tested, education and behavioral measures showed they could be successful in places like Thailand (Cohen 1995) and Kenya (Nowak 1995), as well as in the United States. Nevertheless, no one enforced equipoise standards in places like Thailand or Africa.

There were also fundamental scientific problems with testing vaccine candidates in Africa. The candidate vaccines in preparation in the United States were genetically engineered from American and European strains of HIV (Barnes 1988; Palca 1991a; Cohen 1994a), but planned testing would take place in populations facing entirely different strains of the disease. Jose Esparza, WHO's head of AIDS vaccine development, recognized American vaccine manufacturers' reluctance to develop vaccines designed specifically for the likely test populations in places like Brazil, Uganda, Rwanda, and Thailand: "there's a need here to encourage manufacturers to make strain-specific vaccines" (Cohen 1993f, 981). Along with the ethical problems raised by a vaccine candidate designed for use with a different population than the one on which it was to be tested (a violation of the justice standard), the vaccines that had been developed using American strains of HIV were going to be tested in a population that did not carry the American strains of HIV. Despite evidence for different disease epidemiologies, modes of transmission (Brun-Vézinet, Rouzioux, et al. 1984; Norman 1985b; Linke 1986; Burton 1986), and very different and much more diverse group of HIV strains than in the United States (Benn, Rutledge, et al. 1985), researchers retained their enthusiasm for these Phase III trial sites. The narrative expectation for a successful vaccine doubtless helped the market to retain its primacy, despite the contradictions: "Vaccine manufacturers have little interest in tailoring vaccines specifically for these countries—which have different strains of HIV—when the market is uncertain" (Cohen 1993f).

Even if most of the trials being done in Africa were, in fact, "directed at finding ways to slow Africa's AIDS epidemic" (Nowak 1995, 1333), the vaccine trials had little prospect for any kind of success: they were genetically engineered for the wrong strains of HIV in the test populations. The trials were not designed to develop vaccines for use in Africa, and because of the mismatch between American and African strains of HIV, such trials would have little likelihood of producing vaccines for use anywhere else, either. The correct population to test a vaccine candidate engineered on the basis of American strains of HIV would be a population in which those strains were dominant (inaccessible Americans protected by ethical rules). Proceeding with such trials hardly represented sound science, or even anything like good business planning, and yet the sequence of events described by the narrative seemed to grind inexorably onward, irrespective of the ethical and methodological problems.

The same NIAID decision that turned down the $20 million plan for vaccine trials in the United States "stressed that current tests on any potential AIDS vaccines should continue and that the present decision should not impede efficacy trials in other, harder hit countries, several of which hope to launch real-world tests soon" (Cohen 1994c, 1839). Consultants to WHO agreed, saying that the kinds of trials that were ruled out by NIH shouldn't be ruled out in countries suffering with the epidemic, reasoning that "a more empirical, trial-and-error approach is warranted in parts of the world that are harder hit by HIV than the

United States" (Holden 1994a, 735). This double standard based on the severity of the epidemic implied on the one hand that the epidemic in the United States had abated sufficiently to reduce the immediate need for a vaccine there. On the other hand, high rates of transmission became a justification for trials in places like Africa as part of a plan for halting the raging epidemic there, though the reason for aborting the American-based trials had been the lack of scientific evidence of efficacy, not the abatement of the epidemic. These contradictory rationales for conducting tests outside the United States also conflated methodological requirements for a rigorous trial with the usefulness of such a trial in an affected population; the two are not related.

Linking vaccine research to a remedy for epidemics extended the narrative of vaccination to include even the process of discovering a vaccine as part of the story's happy ending. It suggests that participation in vaccine research would confer benefits on the participating population. This is a mistake that participants in drug trials often make (Applebaum, Roth, et al. 1987), but conducting research offered little immediate help for the people living with high rates of HIV transmission. Vaccine trials, in and of themselves, provide no protection for research subjects, and are not a public health measure. The purpose of the field trial is to determine a vaccine candidate's ability to confer protection from disease in a real-world situation, but trials do not provide medical or other aid to populations used in studies. On the contrary, researchers' reluctance to include behavioral counseling in their trial protocols set up a situation in which medical personnel would, by withholding information that could help subjects prevent infection, give tacit sanction to practices that had high risks for transmission. The authority of the "white coat" of medicine often conveys a message of helpfulness that is not justified in the research context (Christakis 1988). This has been called the "therapeutic misconception," in which subjects will often interpret, even if it requires distortion, the information they receive as part of informed consent disclosures to maintain the view—obviously based on their wishes—that every aspect of the research project to which they have consented was designed to benefit them directly (Applebaum, Roth, et al. 1987, 20).

Vaccine trials must prioritize continued high rates of infection (in order to discover a preventive), over behavioral counseling, if they are going to produce scientifically valid information about the effectiveness of the vaccine candidates; when there are no alternative preventives, such research risks subjects' continued health. In the planning for vaccine trials in the early 1990s, the desirability of a vaccine—whether in terms of an "answer" to the epidemic or simply in terms of bringing a successful product to market in the United States and Europe—seems to have won out over ethical concerns. This is even more remarkable (but not surprising) as ethical rules insist that the vulnerability of a population suffering epidemic disease should trigger higher ethical thresholds for their participation in vaccine trials.

▇ A Resilient and Powerful Narrative

In 1996 researchers discovered a combination of protease and reverse transcriptase inhibitors that could effectively prevent HIV from replicating in infected people, and reduce their "viral load" to the point that HIV became almost undetectable (Cohen 1996). Though the world greeted this news with enthusiasm and relief, the news did not shake Americans' faith in vaccines as a necessary response to the epidemic. Just as researchers were confirming the positive effects of the drug "cocktails" in 1997, President Clinton made a speech calling for a "new national goal for science": an AIDS vaccine (Mitchell 1997). Since then, different kinds of AIDS vaccine trials have been initiated and some completed, though none has shown any efficacy. Then, as now, most researchers pursuing a vaccine sincerely believe that it holds the key to stopping the epidemic. As one research report put it, "alterations in the life-styles of certain high-risk groups may help to reduce the spread of the disease, but the development of a reliable vaccine against the AIDS retrovirus would be more effective in arresting the current epidemic" (Lasky, Groopman, et al. 1986, 209). There was no evidence to support this contention then, and some statistical models had shown that apposite condom use had a better chance of stopping the spread of the disease than a vaccine[10] (Pinkerton and Abramson 1993).

To conform to the narrative, researchers preferred a therapeutic vaccine to no vaccine or to reliance on behavioral preventives (even if they worked). One NIAID researcher explained the shift from preventive to therapeutic vaccines: "If sterilizing immunity is the way a vaccine is going to work, we should put all our money into condom distribution" (Cohen 1993g, 1820). Clearly, the intent was not to argue for condoms. Researchers would not abandon an HIV/AIDS vaccine because a preventive vaccine was not feasible; that would mean abandoning the vaccine narrative. Condom distribution, here presented as a sarcastic alternative to a vaccine, was in fact a real and effective strategy to prevent the spread of HIV. There is still no "end" to the HIV/AIDS chapter in the vaccine narrative. Though no Phase III vaccine trials were carried out between 1981 and 1996, when the effective drug cocktails became available, efforts and enthusiasm for a vaccine continued[11] (Walgate 2003; Flynn, Forthal, et al. 2005). Through all the changes that HIV and AIDS wrought in American society, the expectations surrounding a vaccine solution has remained remarkably unaffected. More than surviving the HIV/AIDS epidemic and the failure of vaccine efforts to combat it, the vaccine narrative remains as strong and persuasive as ever.

In the uneasy equilibrium between ethical rules and methodological efficiency, ethics increasingly prevail—we prefer to err on the side of subjects' safety and autonomy. By contrast, in the search for an HIV/AIDS vaccine, the imperative to produce a vaccine succeeded, at least in the short term, in shifting that balance back in favor of putatively more effective tests and experiments at the cost of some hard-won and easily abused subject rights (informed consent, equipoise, justice). Throughout the first fifteen years of the HIV/AIDS epidemic, vaccines held a prominent and at times dominant place among hoped-for solutions to the disease. In fact, when viewed through the professional literature in which scientists, policymakers, and physicians justified their actions and stated their goals, the vaccine narrative seems to be the only explanation for continued insistence that a vaccine could prevail against such a disease in such an epidemiological, social, and scientific situation. The course of HIV/AIDS vaccine research efforts through 1996 suggests that the promise of an effective vaccine could overwhelm established rules of ethical conduct, and, in important ways, eclipse even aspects of the same established scientific research methods that scientific medicine points to as its provenance.

Of course, within the United States, ethical rules have remained in force, and the inclination to export the risks of HIV/AIDS vaccine testing did not go without a spirited response from within the research community (Cohen 2001). Though changes since 1996 have brought global HIV/AIDS vaccine trials into closer compliance with recognized ethical standards for research on human subjects, attempts to use non-Western populations in other kinds of HIV/AIDS prevention trials occasionally resurface. When American researchers began testing a drug they hoped might prevent HIV infection in southeast Asia (tenofovir—not a vaccine), ACT-UP Paris helped Cambodian prostitutes organize concerted protests to halt the trials there and in Cameroon (Lee 2005). Here AIDS activists were supporting better science and ethics, in light of the alternatives to a preventive. Unlike many other diseases for which researchers have sought vaccines (like the modern archetype, polio), the HIV/AIDS epidemic had alternative preventives.

Education and behavior modification achieved surprising but well-documented successes as practical methods for preventing transmission. This makes it possible to consider vaccination initiatives in a comparative context (which could not be done for polio), most clearly around the issue of equipoise. Laboratory, germ-theory based options were the clearly preferred responses, both culturally and within the health professions, but the initial lack of interest and funding for AIDS created a void that allowed activists and others the space to consider (because they had no choice) other options. As soon as it became clear that AIDS was sexually transmissible, behavioral measures could help; such strategies did not depend on isolating the specific cause of AIDS. These methods (which harkened back to pre-germ theory measures for contending with infectious disease) were so successful that populations that adopted them actually achieved transmission rates too low for vaccine trials. Including counseling about these methods in vaccine trials also threatened to render the trials moot—with effective behavior counseling, infection rates would plummet. Despite the lethality of the disease, the social difficulties of dealing with a sexually transmitted disease and the existence of a viable alternative preventive, Americans kept looking to and hoping for a vaccine to solve the entire range of problems (Barnes 1988).

One consistently remarkable aspect of the search for an HIV/AIDS vaccine was that it seemed to bear so little recognition of the reality of the situation. Faced with a disease transmitted by sex and blood (private behaviors), vaccine researchers and policymakers acted as if they faced a new version of measles—a casually transmitted disease that had no significant social components. Frustrated by their inability to meet standards for the development of a vaccine (e.g., evidence of efficacy in an animal model), researchers lowered the standards. Discovering that HIV mutated quickly, researchers engineered vaccines based on particular or even rare strains that would have, at best, narrow efficacy. Realizing that a preventive vaccine was unlikely, researchers resurrected therapeutic vaccines to salvage the idea of at least some kind of a vaccine against AIDS. Confronted with thorny and complex ethical obstacles to research, companies, researchers, and regulators looked for places where the ethical rules were less enforceable. Most remarkable of all, researchers were at times willing to begin vaccine trials for candidates that had been engineered from a different strain than existed in the test population, indicating a willingness to compromise the basic premise of the germ theory—that each disease is caused by a unique and specific germ—in the quest for a vaccine.[12] The willingness to undermine the methodological logic of vaccine research suggests the strength of the yearning to produce a vaccine: some researchers, anyway, seemed poised to discard the scientific bases for an HIV/AIDS vaccine in the quest to achieve an HIV/AIDS vaccine. Complaints about the unprofitability of vaccines, the high costs and concerns about liability all militated against producing an HIV/AIDS vaccine. Dedication to a vaccine solution—the climax of the story—seemed poised to throw the scientific method out the window.

The corollary of a strong cultural narrative of vaccines, with its ability to guide expectations and behaviors, is the power that vaccine supporters carry into their endeavors because they align themselves with the narrative. Vaccines can serve important economic, professional, and cultural interests. Regardless of their intentions (which may depend on the situation), vaccine developers are an integrated part of what Stanley Wohl (1984) called the "medical industrial complex." In the entrepreneurial climate of American medical research that has prevailed since the 1980s, any company involved in producing an HIV/AIDS vaccine candidate stood to earn enormous profits and world renown if successful in Phase III trials, and to sustain potentially devastating losses if it failed—regardless of the ultimate effect on the epidemic. Moreover, the idea of an HIV/AIDS vaccine, however elusive or unlikely, continued to extend and reaffirm faith in vaccines as our "solution" to the problem of other infectious diseases.

The prospect of professional standing and profits from a successful HIV/AIDS vaccine must form part of the explanation for the continued interest in vaccine research. The technical difficulties involved in developing an HIV/AIDS vaccine were not necessarily a discouragement to researchers, because AIDS was "also scientifically exciting" and its study promised to produce important knowledge about the human immune system in general (Kolata 1983, 436). In arguing for a vaccine response to HIV/AIDS, mainstream researchers both in government and at private companies stood to benefit, as research dollars flowed to them along with the possibility of fame and lucrative vaccine patents. Those without vested interests in the success or failure of vaccines took what appears, at least in retrospect, to be a more disinterested view. The editors of *Science* magazine commented as early as 1986 that, especially given that a vaccine might mean waiting as long as a decade, "our most powerful tools in the next few years will be information, education, and prevention campaigns. To some scientists these terms may sound abstract, even vacuous—but not to public health professionals or social scientists" (Jenness 1986, 825). This attitude made little impact on the search for a vaccine. The course of vaccine initiatives then beginning in the mid-1980s suggests that the prospects of an effective vaccine were so remote, and the steps taken towards developing an effective vaccine candidate sufficiently flawed, as to make a viable vaccine outcome a remote possibility, at best. But to hear researchers tell it, vaccines would be a panacea for HIV/AIDS, or at any rate, as Jonas Salk put it, "the best hope" (Salk, Bretscher, et al. 1993, 1270).

Some of these attitudes can be understood as part of normal human behavior—strivings for profit and fame, the desire to do good or to save lives. What unifies and motivates them here is the underlying certitude that pervades the literature that never had to be explained or justified: a vaccine held the key. Without broad cultural acceptance of vaccination as the natural and best solution to infectious disease, we would not have such faith that the story we know and accept about vaccines can apply equally to HIV/AIDS; there would have been little hope for profits or professional advancement, and there would not have been much budgetary support from government and policymakers. Perhaps it was easier to bend ethical rules and weaken established evidentiary standards than to acknowledge that a vaccine might not be the answer to the HIV/AIDS crisis. It is difficult to escape the irony that in the search for an HIV/AIDS vaccine, researchers began to erode the very scientific standards that supply the empirical basis for vaccination in the first place. The vaccine solution may still seem to us like the perfect response to HIV and AIDS, but we need to be reflective enough to ask why that is so, given that even strong belief does not necessarily transform a powerful cultural narrative into a practical or feasible response to an epidemic.

Conclusion

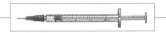

*The bottom line is that vaccines
are good and disease is bad.*

—L. D. Frenkel
and K. Nielsen (2003)

Vaccines Are Essential

In early October of 2004, concerns about contamination led the British government to shut down Chiron Corporation's production facility in the United Kingdom that made flu vaccines for the United States. Suddenly and unexpectedly, it looked as if the United States would have many fewer doses of the vaccine than anticipated, and American public health agencies scrambled to ensure that enough of the vaccine would be available to protect vulnerable populations. Small stocks of an alternative nasal-spray vaccine preparation were considered for use instead of the Chiron vaccine, and the only other company licensed to produce flu vaccine for the United States promised to step up production by an additional million or so doses. Even so, the best projections suggested that the United States would not be able to satisfy the anticipated need; instead of 100 million doses, only 54 million would be available.

Caught between the sudden shortage and the pressing needs of the impending flu season, public health officials, hospitals, and other health institutions presented the public with a "don't worry" crisis. On the one hand, the message was that the flu threat was real and the vaccine was essential; an epidemic could devastate those most vulnerable: the elderly, the sick and the very young. This meant that supplies would be allocated on the basis of careful prioritization of need; those outside the priority groups were "asked to forego or defer vaccination" (CDCP 2004b). The shortage would therefore require serious sacrifice by large numbers of people. At the same time, the message reassured the public that there was no need to panic, that halving the available supply did not pose any special risks. Suggestions for those not on the priority vaccine list took a page from the pre-germ theory era precautions: to stay away from sick people, to cover sneezes and coughs, and to stay home from work or school when sick (Thompson 2004).

As the 2004–2005 flu season proceeded, however, the feared public health calamity failed to materialize. Aside from isolated stories of price gouging and profiteering by individual vaccine purveyors and the occasional physician, the flu vaccine shortage turned out to be neither an administrative nor a health crisis. By the middle of the flu season, the shortage appeared to have turned into a kind of surplus—not because of new stocks of additional doses, but because people were not getting themselves vaccinated (Manier 2004). Moreover, while the Centers for Disease Control and Prevention estimates that with adequate vaccine stocks seasonal flu typically causes about 36,000 deaths and more than 200,000 hospitalizations each year (CDCP 2004a), the 2004–2005 season appears to have been about average when compared to the previous four flu seasons (CDCP 2005; Fukuda 2005). In fact, the death rate from the flu was as good as or better than the two previous seasons. In this real-world experiment, a drastic vaccine shortage failed to produce any new public health crisis, under conditions that saw vaccination rates as low as thirty-five percent among the highest priority groups (Stein 2004).

Coming in the month before a closely contested presidential election and in the middle of heightened concerns about bio-terror attacks, the flu vaccine shortage became a political football. The Bush administration received sustained criticism for its failure to anticipate something as simple as a flu vaccine shortage, especially given the post-9/11 context and fears about biological weapons in the hands of terrorists (e.g., James 2004; Kuttner 2004; Nesmith and McKenna 2004). Less partisan public comments focused on the imprudence of relying on so few suppliers for such a crucial resource, and the fact that when the Chiron vaccine plant shut down, it was a foreign government's decision—a decision believed crucial to the health and well-being of American citizens—that cut the supply (NYT 2004). The fear that the United States was unprepared for something as routine as seasonal flu triggered reflections on the nature of the vaccine infrastructure, the reasons for its condition, and ways to fix it. This broader public discussion about the state of vaccine production did not offer a good prognosis:

> "The vaccine infrastructure is frail," said Dr. Paul A. Offit, chief of infectious diseases at Children's Hospital of Philadelphia. Dr. Offit said that 7 of the 12 pediatric vaccines were made by a single manufacturer and that there had been shortages at one time or another

of nine of them since 1998. One reason is that vaccines are not that profitable to drug companies. (Pollack 2004)

Profitability, previously rarely mentioned in the context of vaccination, became a common refrain in public discussions to explain both the flu shortage and general problems with vaccine supply. One op-ed columnist argued that

> Flu vaccine should be an attractive product for manufacturers. . . . but, like virtually all other vaccines, it isn't profitable. And that has discouraged vaccine development to the point that supplies of many lifesaving vaccines are in jeopardy. The fundamental problem is that government policies discourage companies from investing aggressively to develop new vaccines. (Miller 2004)

Similar arguments came from pharmaceutical companies, who had with less fanfare been insisting for some time that vaccines were difficult to develop and produce and carried little expectation of profit; they called such biologics "orphan drugs."

In 1998, Donald Francis, Randy Shilts's heroic researcher in *And the Band Played On*, was an AIDS vaccine researcher with Genentech Corporation when he voiced concerns about the failure to embrace the virtues of preventive vaccination in terms less commercial, but still conveying the sense that vaccines had somehow lost the respect they deserved:

> Vaccines by and large, I think, in—more so—I've worked a lot in the developing world. More so in industrial societies interestingly—don't always have the value that they should have. We want the magic bullet, the liver-heart-lung transplant, and don't think about the simple way of just prevention in the first place. . . . [I]t's not been given a priority by our society. (Francis 1998, 12)

This characterization of vaccines as a victim of neglect, as an "orphan drug," creates an interesting and powerful metaphor that turns our society into the unfeeling orphanage that cannot find resources to care properly for something as valuable as vaccines.

The orphan-drug metaphor implies that vaccines (which we all acknowledge have saved us from deadly epidemics, protected our children from dangerous scourges, and pushed infectious diseases off the mortality tables) deserve better treatment; vaccines should not be left to languish without support or resources, as if they were an elective luxury. Given the perceived threats posed by the flu vaccine shortage—to the public health in general, to the most vulnerable members of society, as well as to homeland security and national defense—

the idea of vaccines as mistreated orphans quickly became part of the public discussions about vaccines. This metaphor and its associated meanings gained currency as the discourse broadened into issues about the "frailty" of vaccine production. It simultaneously clarified and acknowledged a new role for profit in our cultural narrative of vaccination, with the corporation as the willing but under-resourced foster parent to the orphan vaccines.

Narratives Change

Narratives tell stories that help us frame and understand our reality; they need not be true stories. The nature of cultural narratives, as Patricia Ewick and Susan Silbey (2003) argue, is to take an event and turn it into a story. The earliest narratives about vaccines and vaccination came to us out of the 1790s, telling of Edward Jenner's discovery of smallpox vaccine and how it heralded the end not only of smallpox, but of disease and perhaps death itself. Jenner's innovative use of cowpox to protect against smallpox has changed over the decades into a story of genius and simplicity, in which geniuses—like Jenner—devote themselves to discovering ways for our bodies to self-protect, with a little help. That help, the result of serendipity (as with smallpox) or diligent scientific research (as with polio) is the simplest and most elegant of interventions: the vaccine. Introducing a small quantity of safe matter into our bodies, vaccination confers life-long protection against disease, just as surviving a case of the common cold makes us forever immune to that specific cold virus. The vaccine narrative tells a better story than that, however: vaccines are also equal-opportunity protectors, and because they are so easy and cost effective, they have become central to our society's ability to help people irrespective of their wealth or social standing. Told in this way, vaccines are the quintessential progressive innovation: we all benefit from vaccines, and by their careful and diligent application, we do more than just help ourselves, we share the benefits of scientific discovery with the least fortunate while putting deadly diseases on the road to eradication.

The modern vaccine narrative, as I have argued in the preceding chapters, grew out of the institutions and interests supportive of preventive vaccination in each of the historical periods, beginning in the 1720s, with smallpox inoculation in Boston. Smallpox vaccination followed around 1800, and was bolstered by publicity about rabies vaccine in the 1880s. In the 1920s, successes with diphtheria mass vaccination turned doctors and public health officials into full supporters.

For average Americans, vaccines achieved their prominence during the Salk polio vaccine trials in the mid-1950s. Polio vaccine's modern version of the narrative overrode the earlier controversies and problems of smallpox vaccine (which sometimes killed people) with a clear and positive story that has been highly durable, not least because of the successes of other vaccine initiatives and the close association with scientific medicine and public health. But it also benefited from the simplicity and cultural consonance of its elements: to combat an infectious disease, selfless physician-researchers use their initiative and know-how to (1) discover the responsible microbe; (2) develop a preventive vaccine that protects everyone; (3) obtain government and professional sponsorship for mandatory mass vaccination campaigns (despite ignorant opposition); and (4) proceed towards eradication of the disease in the United States, and ultimately the world. The same narrative has served for all kinds of diseases, across a wide range of factors, such as mortality rates, adverse reactions, modes of transmission, and practical concerns about implementation, to name a few. Over the last century, different groups have questioned or opposed vaccination, sometimes with scientific standing and other times without any seeming rational basis, and the dominant narrative has by and large held firm and even triumphed. That is not to say that *vaccines* have triumphed (viz. the lack of attention to the "frailty" of the institutions of production), but the main elements of the narrative we tell about them have remained largely intact.

Though resilient in the face of most contrary facts or interpretations, and enduring over many decades, cultural narratives are not immutable. They are, at least theoretically, infinitely mutable. Like the children's game of telephone, their existence is largely discursive, and relies on the retelling of stories for the plot of the narrative to survive. Social power and authority, access to media and publicity, as well as cultural and practical resonance (it is certainly reassuring to believe that vaccines do, indeed, protect us from infectious disease) can all be important factors in sustaining any particular narrative. Still, the changing context of the story remains crucially important for our sense of the events narrated; narratives respond to the retelling environment.

The shift from a narrative of vaccination as a pure public beneficence to something understood in the more prosaic context of profit-and-loss statements is particularly interesting because it contravenes one of the central elements of the original story: the selfless and dedicated scientist/researcher who discovers the vaccine. The narrative does not prepare us to expect profit to motivate researchers to find new vaccines; pharmaceutical companies are not characters in the story. Both the stories and the histories agree that Jenner (smallpox), Pasteur (rabies, anthrax), Park (diphtheria), and Salk or Sabin (both polio) were not driven by profit. Of course, most of us know Salk's name, and fame and success have always been important to medical discoveries; but personal glory is different than economic success. Even personal profit is different than the institutional momentum we find in the pharmaceutical industry.

The corollary to the narrative thread that says profit does not motivate vaccine research is that lack of profit should not hinder vaccine development. But recent experiences, and not only with flu vaccines, have shown that at least in this respect, we no longer expect the selfless researcher to play a crucial part in the story: the profit/loss calculation has begun to figure prominently and publicly in our understanding of vaccines. If it is reasonable for vaccine companies to earn a profit making vaccines, it is a short leap to the idea that only profit makes vaccine development and production possible. The underlying narrative remains the same: scientists will develop, test and deploy vaccines that will protect us—and the vaccines remain the true heroes of the story. But as the context has changed, it has increasingly brought medicine into the commercial realm. This is not a minor change in the narrative.

There is an enormous difference between an individual medical hero and a corporate laboratory. Part of the glamour and excitement of the vaccine narrative derives from the heroic inventor/discoverer associated with each vaccine. We cannot help but trust, respect, and revere Jonas Salk, who devoted himself to ridding the world of paralytic polio; but can we feel this way about Merck, Inc., when they produce a vaccine against human papilloma virus (HPV), which promises to eradicate cervical cancer? Here we find one of the functions of a cultural narrative—to present a template for the stories we hear. In this way we can fit the HPV vaccine into the pre-existing vaccine narrative, as we begin to equate the accomplishments of Salk with those of the essentially anonymous team of Merck researchers. We know, after all, how the polio vaccine story goes (epidemics cause death, genius discovers prevention, deployment through mass vaccination saves lives, continued use brings eradication), and so we can simply substitute the HPV vaccine, and we have ready acceptance of the new vaccine—despite enormous differences between the diseases, the vaccines, the populations involved, the politics, and the alternatives to vaccination.

These new and different parts of the narrative are not necessarily incompatible; this is the mutable nature of narrative. Particularly given the advertising industry's consummate skill in adopting and co-opting cultural trends (including narratives) as a way to increase sales and profits, people seem quite willing to accept these minor variations in the vaccine story. Just as the television commercials for clothing shamelessly feature peace signs (which have nothing to do with the clothing), Merck's new television ads use the phrase "tell someone" and images of younger and older women to conflate the women's health movement and mother-daughter relationships with their desire to sell Gardasil, their new HPV vaccine.[1] In a society in which drug companies solicit the public to ask physicians for specific prescription medications, perhaps the idea that corporations are legitimate characters in the story of public health is not so far-fetched.

Over the past fifty years, medical and pubic health research (as well as health care) have become increasingly commercialized, and the attendant changes in the institutions, practices, and structures governing vaccine development have helped create the different context for the narratives we tell about vaccines. When rubella vaccine was being researched in the late 1960s, for example, the role of government was primarily to fund and facilitate the development of an effective rubella vaccine in anticipation of a major epidemic; regulators were all-but-invisible partners speeding approval of vaccines. By the time that serious efforts were underway to develop an HIV/AIDS vaccine in the 1990s, the relationship between government and corporate research entities had changed dramatically. When the $20 million congressional appropriation for HIV/AIDS vaccine research became available in 1991, the National Institute of Allergy and Infectious Diseases (NIAID) intervened to prevent vaccine companies from using the money on projects that lacked a sound scientific basis.

Today, faced with threats of anthrax and smallpox terror scares, corporate producers want "fast-track" approval for their products (which typically involves reduced clinical testing) and at least some immunity from liability claims, should there be any adverse effects of the vaccines. Such changes and new relationships have fostered a slow-but-sure change in our understandings of vaccination. While most elements of the vaccine narrative have persisted, to judge by the response to the flu vaccine shortage, we now seem to accept vaccination as part of a commercial enterprise, with government serving—at best—as a funding source and potential watchdog.

In fact, considering vaccines to be "orphan drugs" reshuffles the characters in the vaccine narrative. It relies on and perhaps even strengthens our faith in vaccines, because it asks us to direct our complaints at the government, not the researchers, drug corporations, or the vaccines themselves. In a similar way, profit introduces a new motivation but not a new plot into the vaccine story; it replaces the old-style heroes with human faces (Jenner, Pasteur, Salk) with corporations developing profitable drugs (the vaccines themselves). Vaccines, which were our staunch protectors, now are themselves vulnerable orphans in need of protection. As one commentator put it, the flu vaccine shortage in 2004–2005 came about because vaccines are orphans, and they are orphans because of the government:

> The US government has crippled the vaccine industry. . . . Now, only four companies [manufacture childhood vaccines] . . . because our government has destroyed all the incentives. . . . Strict screening for safety by the FDA costs lots of time and money. Then, there's unchecked legal action. . . . Decades of disastrous vaccine policy have left us unprepared. (Pipes 2005)

This argument comes almost verbatim from arguments made less publicly by pharmaceutical companies in general since at least the 1980s. It relies on our acceptance of the narrative that vaccines are so important that society should forego a host of established safety and procedural policies and practices to obtain them: drug companies want to produce vaccines, and government (here represented by the FDA) stands in the way. According to this formulation, in order to help rescue vaccines from the orphanage, we need to abandon "strict screening for safety" at the same time that we need to "check" legal action (that is, deny people who suffer adverse effects from unsafe vaccines the right to sue for damages, or simply put, protect pharmaceutical companies' profits from legal action against them by people harmed by their profitable drugs). These stances serve to solidify the importance of vaccines and the orphan-drug reputation for vaccines. They also use aspects of the narrative as a lever to obtain legal and regulatory changes to boost profits for drug companies.

Drug manufacturing is an enormously profitable business. In fact, the calls to change the safety and other constraints on vaccine production as a way to make them cost-effective for manufacturers imply that vaccines today are as important and necessary for continued public health as they were during the times when smallpox, cholera, and diphtheria epidemics were a regular feature of life and the biggest causes of infant mortality were common infectious diseases.[2] The recent flu vaccine shortage, however, showed that at least in that year, the absence of flu vaccine did not make much difference. We accept that vaccines were central to the eradication of smallpox and polio, but that does not mean that contemporary vaccines continue to perform the same role that they did in decades past. It is true that the seasonal flu could easily be much worse in another year, and in preparation for that situation, a good supply of effective vaccine can be expected to play an important part of the overall strategy to save lives. Similarly, an effective vaccine would be essential during an avian flu pandemic. But what is most striking about the 2004–2005 flu vaccine shortage is the way it spurred public discussions about the ways to guarantee better access to vaccines based on the benefits vaccines confer, but missed the evidence that—again, if only for that year—the absence of vaccine made little difference to flu morbidity or mortality rates. That alone suggests that we continue to accept vaccines and vaccination as a fundamentally positive and necessary measure: this basic aspect of the plot, at least, remains intact. Reading the accounts of the flu shortage, it becomes obvious that almost no one "saw" the other side of the cost/benefit analysis—that although flu vaccine does confer protection against infection, its absence did not produce appreciable costs.

Don't Panic

The current cultural narrative about vaccines includes heroes (scientists, vaccines themselves—maybe corporations) and villains (anti-vaccinationists, unscrupulous parents who withhold vaccines from their kids, an over-regulating government) but leaves no room for vaccines that may not be so essential to the population's continued good health. Instead, the narrative portrays all vaccines as life-savers—as essential, as necessary. In fact, calling something a vaccine confers a status that almost automatically commands respect as an effective preventive. As the experience with the flu shortage suggests, vaccines, though typically highly effective in conferring immunity, may not always be as necessary in the particular epidemiological context as the narrative suggests (just as vaccination's heroes may not have been the selfless altruists the narrative makes them out to be[3] and the "villains" who oppose vaccination may not be evil-doers). These ideas about vaccination make many people very nervous—not on account of their veracity, but because they may undermine the faith in vaccines that is so important to compliance with vaccination programs, on which, indeed, lives may depend. Whether protecting girls against cervical cancer with the new HPV vaccine (Henican 2007) or saving lives by doing the right thing and getting a flu vaccine (Allen 2007), we continue to believe that vaccines are essential to our continued good health.

The worst-case scenario for vaccine failure, of course, involves not seasonal flu, but a deadly avian flu pandemic or a bio-terrorist attack using anthrax or smallpox. In such cases, if there isn't enough vaccine, how will people (and institutions) react to rationing programs? Many viewed the 2004–2005 flu vaccine shortage as a real-world dry run that tested national coordination of rationed vaccine. The consensus evaluation of the outcome of that experience with a vaccine shortage seems to have been reassuring: no significant rioting, price-gouging, or profiteering; people behaved in an orderly and organized way.

Yet the vaccine narrative's promise that vaccines can and will save us creates an entirely different order of problems: The traditional version of the narrative would rely on American ingenuity and creativity (the humble genius) to come up with a "Manhattan project" type initiative to solve the problem. The new version of the narrative, which seems to dominate the current public discussions, asks for something very different: drug companies need to have a freer hand in producing vaccines, simply because when vaccines become "orphans" Americans' safety suffers. That new story, in turn, is predicated on the idea of the vaccine as the true hero of the story: the vaccine (whether invented by the next Jonas Salk or hatched in the corporate labs of a multinational pharmaceutical company) will, indeed, save us from the flu, or the smallpox attack.

Of course most vaccines are simply routine (though the same narrative applies to them), and we also rely on vaccines to protect us against generally non-lethal disease—like mumps. Mumps makes a good example of the resilience of the narrative in the face of some recent complicating facts: a relatively innocuous childhood disease, mumps is implicated in sterility among men who contract it as adults. An outbreak (more than 2500 verified cases) of mumps in the Midwest seemed to suggest that mumps vaccine is far less effective than long believed: though the disease appeared in greater proportions among the unvaccinated, many of the children who caught the disease had been fully vaccinated (Grady 2006b). Despite the failure to guarantee immunity to mumps (the narrative tells about vaccines providing complete protection), the public response to the outbreak from health professionals might have come straight out of a mayoral proclamation about smallpox or diphtheria vaccine in the 1930s:

> The basic advice is this, said Thomas T. Rubio, professor of pediatrics in the infectious disease division at Georgetown University Hospital: Verify that children have received two MMR (measles, mumps, rubella) vaccinations. He also said most adults who have not had both injections should consider getting one now. One more thing: Don't panic. (Edwards 2006)

The injunction not to panic is well placed, because the failure of a vaccine to protect sounds an alarm among everyday people and also among those charged with the job of making sure everyone gets vaccinated, but for different reasons.

For average Americans, a less-than-perfect vaccine raises questions about adverse effects and the attendant personal risks and benefits of compliance (or non-compliance) with mass vaccination policies. For vaccine proponents, anything less than complete and unilateral support for vaccination programs seems to engender just the reaction that health professionals warn lay people not to have: panic. Vaccine proponents sometimes seem more concerned about deviations from the narrative (that might lower compliance with vaccination rules) than with real changes in the structure of vaccination production.

The Nature of Narratives and the Future of the Vaccine Narrative

Despite claims that vaccines have become too expensive to research, not profitable enough to produce, and an unappreciated and money-losing public service that drug companies provide to the public, new vaccines continue to appear. In 2006, the American Academy of Pediatrics website reported that fourteen new vaccines were either awaiting FDA approval or under consideration for expanded use. In addition to recent vaccines against Lyme disease and chicken pox, ongoing research continues into new vaccines designed to protect people against rotavirus, pneumococcus bacteria, and meningitis; "booster" vaccines against pertussis and chicken pox (including a therapeutic vaccine against shingles); and new combinations of existing (or slightly modified) vaccines. Between 1983 and 2002 (the most recent update), the number of vaccines recommended by the government's Advisory Committee on Immunization Practices for small children increased from ten shots to protect against seven diseases to twenty-eight different injections for fifteen different diseases (CDCP 1983, 2002). This level of productivity suggests that there continues to be an active vaccine industry. The issues of profitability are complicated, and the analysis of drug companies' finances is far beyond the scope of this book, but perhaps changes in the meaning of "reasonable profit" have legitimated the expectation of billion-dollar drug profits.[4]

If our faith in the worthiness of vaccines is, at least in part, a social and historical construct that maintains and supports itself through narratives, what does this mean? The greatest concern is that questioning vaccines' positivistic provenance will lead to decreasing compliance. At a different level, the very idea that our faith in vaccines derives from something like a cultural narrative threatens to undermine the place of rationality and reason. Vaccines originally earned such widespread support because of strong empirical evidence, and they remain closely associated with scientism and the laboratory (as any medical or public health journal will confirm). But if the narrative of vaccines has been a potent force for convincing average people to believe in and comply with vaccine policy (independent of laboratory reports or expert knowledge), then examining that narrative may appear to threaten vaccine compliance. The notion that vaccination's benefits are "part of a story" is a subversive and dangerous idea. At the same time, the scientific method—to which sociologists at some level subscribe—requires us to look at all the evidence, even (or especially) if it threatens to undermine deeply held beliefs about what is right. Understanding how narratives work, and the vaccine narrative is only one example of a powerful cultural narrative, is as much an obligation for sociologists as understanding how avian flu works is for health professionals.

When we hear deviations from a cultural narrative, we have difficulty accepting them. This makes narratives a lot like scientific (or cultural) paradigms. The difference between a narrative and a paradigm (or an ideology, or a belief system) is simply that narratives tell a story—a predictable series of events, with certain kinds of "characters" and with a known plot. Vaccines have become the paradigmatic strategy to solve problems of health. Investigating the narrative that supports that paradigm makes it necessary to question the extent to which their continued dominance in the general culture derives from empirical evidence about their efficacy and other objective sources of factual information. It seems that strong support from the cultural narrative that informs our everyday understanding of vaccines may have been crucial to their continued prominence, despite the decline (from vaccination or other causes) of most infectious disease.[5]

To judge by the continued production of new and potentially profitable vaccines, the cultural provenance of vaccines remains quite strong, despite reports of institutional "frailty." In fact, the claims for changes in the regulation of vaccine production rely heavily on our understanding of vaccines that comes from the narrative. Vaccines might be strengthened by closer monitoring of safety concerns, and a more critical look at the need for a vaccine in each individual case. This would involve a conscious anticipation of the claims of vaccine critics, as well as recognition of the extent to which vaccines' reputation relies on a successful narrative, rather than simply on an inherently successful and easily transposable technology. Too often, we see vaccines as so important a step to eradicating disease and even as an end in themselves that we may become careless of possible negative ramifications or dismissive of viable alternatives.

Approving for use or even mandating a new or additional vaccine does not typically ask much of the general population. The bureaucratic, ideological, and narrative structures are already in place. One more vaccine disturbs the status quo very little in the way of behavioral changes, and, as an Institute of Medicine Report (IOM 1988a) found, does not present elected members the polity with the problem of "offending constituents"—as condom programs, early sex education, and open discussions of health and private behaviors sometimes do. This helps explain the absence of vaccine initiatives against diseases like syphilis and gonorrhea and the anomalous controversy around mandatory HPV vaccination—HPV is sexually transmitted (Hart 2007). The accumulated burden of numerous vaccinations, however, may have their price. Recent news reports suggest that despite record-high compliance rates, parents of young children—that large group of people who accept the narrative, but are not committed to it with the same strength as health professionals—may be reaching their tolerance limit for new vaccines (Connolly 2000).

We see numerous examples in American life today of an expectation for a "quick fix" that will eliminate the need for careful, sometimes tedious behavioral changes. This is not necessarily bad, but it is worth noting, especially to the extent that such expectations have reached into our medical policymaking. The fact remains that the historical appearance of vaccines probably did reduce demands from progressive public health advocates for better housing, fresh air, a healthful diet, and good working conditions. It was easier to institute mass diphtheria vaccination than to improve slum living conditions. And today it is "easier" to imagine an HIV/AIDS vaccine than to achieve meaningful sex education or needle exchange programs. Better yet, vaccines should protect us from all the new (and old) diseases. Tina Rosenberg spoke to this recently in a piece in the *New York Times* magazine:

> Last month, scientists invented the AIDS vaccine. Missed it? Perhaps that's because you were still seeking the vaccine fantasy: the magic bullet, the impenetrable shield that finally pitches this disease into the trash bin, the shot that will end not only the AIDS epidemic but our anxiety about the AIDS epidemic as well. (Rosenberg 2007)

Perhaps we still seek "the vaccine fantasy" because we want and need it. Vaccination, as understood by our cultural narrative, provides just such an "impenetrable shield" to reaffirm our sense that human beings can and will control—defeat, eradicate—disease and death. Whether we like it or not, our feelings about vaccines result from our experience within American culture, and our culture sincerely believes in a narrative that casts vaccination as our rescuer from infectious disease. The extent to which that narrative is a "fantasy" is beyond the scope of this book. Recognizing, understanding, and addressing the power of our cultural narrative of vaccines, however, is crucial to our ability to use vaccines as part of our strategy to contend with disease.

Notes

Introduction

1. Even findings about weaker protection from vaccines usually fail to generate much general interest, as when the news broke that the new chickenpox vaccine is, in fact, much less effective than originally believed (Chaves, Gargiullo, et al. 2007).

2. As this sentence makes obvious, I use the terms vaccine[s] and vaccination almost interchangably. This is intentional. On a stylistic level, it is too cumbersome always to write, "vaccines and vaccination" for every instance that involves either or both. In fact, the two words are different sides of the same phenomenon—the vaccine is the thing, while vaccination is the practice of administering vaccines. They are different, but neither exists entirely independent of the other. I try to use the better term in the particular context, but it should never be forgotten that they are interdependent concepts, if not always interchangeable ones.

3. Steeper declines in polio mortality had been recorded in the years leading up to 1920 (McKinlay and McKinlay 1977).

4. Like my use of "vaccines" and "vaccination," I use HIV/AIDS to refer to the virus (HIV), testing positive for HIV, and full-blown AIDS, though when a reference requires more specificity, I will use the other forms individually.

5. Smallpox was highly infectious, often deadly, easily identifiable and appeared in a pattern of epidemics. Almost alone among human infectious disease, smallpox has no non-human vectors (it can only be passed from person to person), is easily identified because of a very specific set of symptoms, and, perhaps most importantly for vaccination, surviving a case of smallpox confers lifelong immunity to it.

6. Perhaps the most succinct characterization of heroic medicine is Martin Kaufman's inventory: "Treatment consisted of bleeding, blistering, vomiting, sweating, purging, and administering massive doses of calomel, often until the patient was at the threshold of acute mercurial poisoning" (Kaufman 1967, 468).

7. Enthusiasm for vaccines as a technology led some researchers, like the immunological pioneer Almoth Wright, to believe that active immunization could be effective not only as a preventive, but as a therapy that would cure a patient even after the disease had been contracted (Worboys 1992, 84). The idea of a "therapeutic vaccine"— of stimulating the immune system after infection—became discredited in the 1930s. In the 1980s and '90s HIV/AIDS vaccine researchers, des-

perate to produce some kind of vaccine, resurrected the idea
(see Chapter 4).

8. That is not to say that the anti-polio campaign was only or even
primarily about publicity. Because polio is caused by a virus, it is
not amenable to antibiotic treatment.

Chapter 1

1. Historians who have tried to understand the success of smallpox
vaccine in the context of the germ theory of disease discovered that
there was little evidence of what Jenner's vaccine contained—it may
even have been a form of inoculation (attenuated smallpox), rather
than anything new (or related to cowpox) at all (Razzell 1977a, 1977b).
2. Diphtheria antitoxin conferred "passive" immunity, because immunity
to the disease relied directly upon and lasted only as long as antitoxin
remained in the body—no more than three or four weeks. "Active"
immunity is a term that health professionals used to describe immunity
that resulted from infection—immunity that derived from the body's
"active" response to disease (or, in the case of diphtheria, "toxin").
Immunity in the modern (early twenty-first century) sense usually
means "active" immunity.
3. This was also part of the movement among regular (allopathic)
medicine practitioners to reorganize medical education, change the
standards of the profession and out-compete all the other health
practitioners—homeopaths, eclectics, midwives, etc. (see Friedson
1973; Markowitz and Rosner 1973; Brown 1979; Starr 1982).
4. This is important for understanding attitudes within the health
professions literature. There was, of course, also a moral imperative
to eradicating germs in the popular culture; see Nancy Tomes (1998)
for an excellent elboration of this popular phenomenon.
5. Out of the more than 50 diphtheria articles directly related to
diphtheria prevention, immunity, and vaccine recorded in the *Index
Medicus* between 1903 and 1930, people associated with the New
York City laboratory authored more than a third.
6. The closing quotation by Goler is from a story included in the article
about a German immigrant family, persuaded by the effectiveness of
the anti-pertussis campaign.
7. The idea of a therapeutic vaccine lost credibility by the 1940s, and
was not revived until in the 1990s by HIV/AIDS researchers desperate
to produce a vaccine (see Chapter 4).

Chapter 2

1. Material in this chapter appeared in a very different form in an article in
the *New England Journal of Public Policy:* Jacob Heller, "Rubella Vac-

cine and Medical Policy-Making: Fetal Rights and Women's Health,"
New England Journal of Public Policy 16, no. 1 (2000):117–38.

2. The March of Dimes Foundation continued to be involved in sponsoring vaccine development research, as well as other medical research related to birth defects. In the early 1960s, for example, before the 1964–65 epidemic, the March of Dimes funded rubella vaccine research with small grants, before it became a major health initiative. Since then it has shifted its support to other kinds of measures to prevent birth defects.

3. Safety concerns do not exist in a vacuum: part of the rationale for rejecting these admittedly dangerous but potentially effective polio vaccines was the concern to "protect public trust in future immunizing agents" (Halpern 2004, 42).

4. Though the lesser-harms standard prevented or curtailed testing in humans of some vaccines, it is less clear that it applied to the evaluation of mass-vaccination campaigns, as subsequent application of rubella vaccine to adult women suggests.

5. See Kristin Luker (1984) for a historical look at American laws and attitudes towards abortion, and John Riddle (1997) for a detailed account of different methods of abortion throughout history.

6. Only since the mid-1960s has the AMA supported legal abortion, arguing that as a medical procedure, abortion should fall under the logic and ethics of patient rights, and that laws should restrict neither the autonomy of the patient nor the options of the physician.

7. Interestingly, in this study the "control" group to which vaccinated women were compared was *also* vaccinated, but was already seropositive for rubella—they showed antibodies to rubella—an unconventional control group. In such a comparison, the two groups "had approximately the same incidence of side effects from vaccination" (Farquar and Corretjer 1969, 268).

8. One of the most prominent rubella researchers at the symposia, Dr. Saul Krugman, later became infamous for violating ethical principles in other research programs. (Rothman and Rothman 1984)

9. The idea of using a vaccine to build herd immunity in a population that is already largely immune raises a number of questions, including whether the 1964–65 epidemic might have been some kind of epidemiological fluke, but also why the mass-vaccination campaign of children was considered so crucial.

Chapter 3

1. Americans have also not typically been impressed by arguments that appear in a form that smacks of "intellectualism" (Hofstadter 1966).

2. This also mirrors some of the tension between American medicine and public health; medicine has typically favored the individual case, the

individual patient. There is also Hippocrates's first ethical principle to "do no harm," which makes no reference to the population, only to the patient.

3. Although there are many similarlties between the tactics and strategies of HIV/AIDS activists and anti-pertussis vaccine activists, including their use of science, the assault on the conclusions of the experts, and grass-roots mobilization efforts, there are also important differences. For example—and unlike the anti-pertussis vaccine movement—the AIDS movement was initially centered within the gay community (an already marginalized group, even within tolerant contexts), and imbued by a corresponding sense of community activism that enabled it to rely on existing organizations (Arno and Feiden 1992); Dissatisfied Parents Together had to develop its own structures and attempt to carve out its own community.

Chapter 4

1. As I mentioned in the Introduction, I use HIV/AIDS to refer to the virus (HIV), testing positive for HIV, and full-blown AIDS, though when a reference requires more specificity, I will use the other forms individually. This avoids confusion but entails some anachronistic use of acronyms. The AIDS virus was originally known by a variety of names, including HTLV-III, LAV, and ARV, until 1986 when an international commission settled on the compromise name of human immunodeficiency virus, or HIV (Marx 1986).

2. Opposition to commonsense prevention programs like free condom distribution, safe-sex education, etc. has frustrated public health advocates who have urged the widespread use of these methods to stem the epidemic. If the history of other sexually transmitted diseases is any indication (Brandt 1985), the short-but-compressed history of HIV/AIDS suggests that social concerns and prejudices about morality and sexual behavior that have influenced venereal disease policies are even more pronounced with AIDS—a preventive mass vaccination program would likely face enormous social opposition.

3. It is difficult to be definitive about the amounts spent on AIDS vaccine research, because such funds are not coordinated, there is any number of ways to categorize funds, and funds can come from a variety of sources (national and local governments, NGO's, corporations, and philanthropies). In the United States (the primary source for HIV/AIDS funds), the NIH has been the main funding source for AIDS vaccine research (CCGHVE 2005). Despite the variety of ways to parse the funding—even within the NIH budget—there was doubtless a steady overall increase in the NIH's annual AIDS funding from about $5,000,000 in 1986 to over $600,000,000 projected in 2007 (Johnson 1998; Nathanson 1999; IAVI 2004; NIH 2006). Over that time, the proportion going towards AIDS vaccines has also increased, from as

little as two percent of NIH's AIDS spending in 1986 to as much as twenty percent projected for 2007 (NIH 2006). Those numbers (and percentages) remain very "soft," however, as the determination of the purposes of research money can be extremely unclear at the time it is spent (no one knows where basic research, for example, will lead). For example, Anthony Fauci, the head of NIAID, reported in 1987 that AIDS vaccine funding constituted about ten percent of NIH's AIDS spending (Cohen 2001), a time when other budget assessments would put vaccine spending closer to two percent of NIH's AIDS research budget (Nathanson 1999).

4. Though this does not mean that vaccine efforts supplanted other, more promising initiatives, it does represent the captivating power of the vaccine solution to the HIV/AIDS crisis.

5. In typical examples, in 1987, Congress voted to promote abstinence education and to withhold funding from educational efforts that were "promoting homosexuality" (Booth 1987). William J. Bennet, Ronald Reagan's Secretary of Education, actively argued for chastity and criticized condom use (Byrne 1989).

6. Sixty years earlier, the prominent vaccine pioneer Almoth Wright had championed therapeutic vaccines. Though he spent the last decades of his life and the better part of his reputation pursuing them as an alternative to other treatments, therapeutic vaccines were ultimately discarded as unworkable (Colebrook 1954; Cope 1966; Worboys 1992).

7. When Harvard University was granted an American patent on a key component of the AIDS virus in 1988 (gp 120, the basis for some of these vaccine candidates), it was deemed lucrative because of its expected usefulness in vaccine development (Sun 1988).

8. The populations in these countries were also largely non-white. This contributed to concerns that racism, rather than science, informed the selection of research sites and research practices, generally (see Sabatier 1988; Christakis 1988).

9. Though NIAID researchers collaborating with Zagury disavowed any involvement with the violation (Barnes 1987a), his collaboration with the National Cancer Institute (NCI, at the time the main arm of the American HIV/AIDS research effort) appeared related to a "mystery break-in" at the laboratory of Dr. Robert Gallo at NCI, who had been credited as co-discoverer of the AIDS virus (Culliton 1990), and Zagury's actions ultimately resulted in a National Institutes of Health (NIH) investigation that rescinded permission for a group of NCI researchers (including Gallo) to collaborate with foreign institutions in France and Zaire (Palca 1991b). Zagury was eventually cleared of ethical violations in vaccine research, though the French government did not investigate the 1987 trials (Dorozynski 1991; Cohen 1992a; Holden 1992), and it was considered by many to be "less than an exoneration" (Holden 1993, 260, 757). Zagury received more negative

press coverage when some of his subsequent vaccine research subjects died (Dorozynski and Anderson 1991; Cohen 1991a).

10. The recent finding confirming circumcision as a barrier to HIV transmission argued that mass circumcision could, if widely applied, serve as a "vaccine" preventive to stop continuing the AIDS epidemic (Muula 2007).

11. Vaccine efforts have continued, though only one vaccine candidate has been fully tested. Commonly known as AIDSVAX, and produced by VaxGen, it was approved for field trials in 1998. It was found to have "no overall protective effect" (Flynn, Forthal, et al. 2005).

12. Some researchers were willing to foreswear the gold standard of efficacy along with the germ theory in favor of hoped-for effectiveness; one researcher argued that it was unimportant to understand why a vaccine worked, as long as it worked (Cohen 1993e).

Conclusion

1. Interestingly, the advertisements on Merck's website contain much more detailed information about both HPV—that it is sexually transmitted, that it *may* be the cause of up to seventy percent of cervical cancers—than about the vaccine, which has shown efficacy against only four strains of HPV, has a list of side effects, and does not confer one hundred percent protection.

2. In 2004, the most common causes of infant mortality were congenital problems, low birth weight, and sudden infant death syndrome; no infectious diseases were reported among the top ten causes (Miniño, Heron, and Smith 2004).

3. Some scholarship has strongly suggested that Pasteur may have been a publicity-crazed appropriator of others' work (Latour 1988) and that Salk was not at all interested in free distribution of his vaccine (Spector 1980) and was highly competitive about beating out his fellow vaccine researchers to get credit for preventing polio; though these claims might be disputed, neither was the selfless genius of the cultural narrative.

4. Reports of adverse effects and lack of efficacy associated with profitable drugs (e.g. Vioxx) suggest the extent to which drugs have become very big business, indeed: public reporting about these problems has focused on the impending profit losses to drug companies and the outcomes of lawsuits for wrongful death, rather than on the profits already earned on sales of ineffective or dangerous drugs. At the same time, advertising by pharmaceutical companies to consumers has ballooned from about $2.5 billion in 2000 (Zarembo 2005) to the neighborhood of $4.5 billion in 2007 (Freudenheim 2007).

5. Thomas Kuhn's groundbreaking work on scientific paradigms (1962), for example, describes something that appears to work in very similar

ways to the idea of a cultural narrative, and the relationship between the two is strong. As Stephen Prickett has described it, you could easily substitute narrative for paradigm: "So conditioned are those within a specific paradigm to expect and look for certain kinds of phenomena, that those that fall outside those expectations, or fail to conform to them, are often literally invisible" (Prickett 2002, 63).

References

AAP, *see* American Academy of Pediatrics.

ACP, *see* American College of Physicians.

Allen, Arthur. 2007. For the Good of the Herd. *The New York Times*, 27 January, p. A25.

Almonte, Paul, and Theresa Desmond. 1991. *The Immune System*. New York: Crestwood House.

Alter, H. J., J. W. Eichberg, H. Masur, W. C. Saxinger, R. Gallo, A. M. Macher, H. C. Lane, and A. S. Fauci. 1984. Transmission of HTLV-III Infection from Human Plasma to Chimpanzees: An Animal Model for AIDS. *Science* 226, no. 4673 (2 November): 549–52.

Altman, Lawrence K. 1982. A New Focus on Whooping Cough Vaccine. *The New York Times*, 8 June, p. C3.

———. 1986. Who Will Volunteer for an AIDS Vaccine? *The New York Times*, 15 April, pp. C1, C7.

———. 2006. Gateses to Finance H.I.V. Vaccine Search. *The New York Times*, 20 July, p. A15.

American Academy of Pediatrics. 1944. *Report by the Council on Therapeutic Procedures for Acute Infectious Diseases and on Biologics*. Evanston, Ill: American Academy of Pediatrics.

———. 1994. *Red Book: Report of the Committee on Infectious Diseases*. 23d ed. Elk Grove Village, Ill.: American Academy of Pediatrics.

American College of Physicians. 1985. *Guide for Adult Immunization*. Philadelphia: American College of Physicians.

———. 1990. *Guide for Adult Immunization*. 2d ed. Philadelphia: American College of Physicians.

———. 1994. *Guide for Adult Immunization*. 3d ed. Philadelphia: American College of Physicians.

Annas, George J., and Michael A. Grodin. 1992. *The Nazi Doctors and the Nuremberg Code*. New York: Oxford University Press.

Applebaum, P., L. Roth, C. Lidz, P. Benson, and W. Winslade. 1987. False Hopes and Best Data: Consent to Research and the Therapeutic Misconception. *Hastings Center Report* 17, no. 2 (April): 20–24.

Arno, Peter S., and Karyn L. Feiden. 1992. *Against the Odds: The Story of AIDS Drug Development, Politics, and Profits*. New York: Harper Collins.

Aronowitz, Robert. 1992. From Myalgic Encephalitis to Yuppie Flu: A History of Chronic Fatigue Syndromes. In *Framing Disease*, edited by Charles E. Rosenberg and Janet Golden, 155–81. New Brunswick, N.J.: Rutgers University Press.

Arthur, L. O., J. W. Bess, Jr., R. C. Sowder II, R. E. Benveniste, D. L. Mann, J. C. Chermann, and L. E. Henderson. 1992. Cellular Proteins Bound to Immunodeficiency Viruses: Implications for Pathogenesis and Vaccines. *Science* 258, no. 5090 (18 December): 1935–38.

Asbury, Carolyn H. 1985. *Orphan Drugs: Medical Versus Market Value.* Lexington, Mass.: Lexington Books.

Atkinson, J. P., and E. J. Bazhaf. 1909–10. The Precipitation of Diphtheria Antitoxin by Means of Precipitins. *Proceedings of the Society for Experimental Biology and Medicine* 7: 148–50.

Baker, Jeffrey P. 2000. Immunization the American Way: 4 Childhood Vaccines. *American Journal of Public Health* 90, no. 2: 199–207.

Balkwill, Fran. 2002. *Germ Zappers.* New York: Cold Spring Harbor Laboratory Press.

Barenberg, L. H. 1918. The Curative and Prophylactic Value of Vaccines in Pertussis. *American Journal of Diseases of Children* 16: 23–29.

Barnes, Deborah M. 1986a. Lethal Actions of the AIDS Virus Debated. *Science* 233, no. 4761 (18 July): 282–83.

———. 1986b. Will an AIDS Vaccine Bankrupt the Company That Makes It? *Science* 233, no. 4768 (5 September): 1035.

———. 1986c. Strategies for an AIDS Vaccine. *Science* 233, no. 4769 (12 September): 1149–53.

———. 1987a. Candidate AIDS Vaccine. *Science* 235, no. 4796 (27 March): 1575.

———. 1987b. Broad Issues Debated at AIDS Vaccine Workshop. *Science* 236, no. 4799 (17 April): 255–57.

———. 1987c. AIDS Vaccine Trial OKed. *Science* 237, no. 4818 (28 August): 973.

———. 1988. Obstacles to an AIDS Vaccine. *Science* 240, no. 4853 (6 May): 719–21.

Barnett, S. W., K. K. Murthy, B. G. Herndier, and J. A. Levy. 1994. An AIDS-Like Condition Induced in Baboons by HIV-2. *Science* 266, no. 5185 (28 October): 642–46.

Barré-Sinoussi, F., J. C. Chermann, F. Rey, M. T. Nugeyre, S. Chamaret, J. Gruest, C. Dauguet, C. Axler-Blin, F. Vézinet-Brun, C. Rouzioux, W. Rozenbaum, and L. Montagnier. 1983. Isolation of T-Lymphotropic Retrovirus from a Patient at Risk for Acquired Immune Deficiency Syndrome (AIDS). *Science* 220, no. 4599 (20 May): 868–71.

Barrie, Herbert. 1983. Campaign of Terror, Letter to Editor. *American Journal of Diseases in Children* 137 (September): 922–33.

Barry, Michele. 1988. Ethical Considerations of Human Investigation in Developing Countries: The AIDS Dilemma. *New England Journal of Medicine* 319, no. 16: 1083–86.

Beasley, R. P. 1970. Dilemmas Presented by the Attenuated Rubella Vaccines. *American Journal of Epidemiology* 92, no. 3: 158–61.

Beauchamp, Tom L., and James F. Childress. 1994. *Principles of Biomedical Ethics*. Oxford: Oxford University Press.

Beecher, Henry Knowles. 1966. Ethics and Clinical Research. *New England Journal of Medicine* 274: 1354–60.

Benn, S., R. Rutledge, T. Folks, J. Gold, L. Baker, J. McCormick, P. Feorino, P. Piot, T. Quinn, and M. Martin. 1985. Genomic Heterogeneity of AIDS Retroviral Isolates from North America and Zaire. *Science* 230, no. 4728 (22 November): 949–51.

Berkeley, Seth. 2001. AIDS Vaccine. *All Things Considered*. National Public Radio, 13 March (search NPR web site at *http://search.npr.org*).

Berkow, Robert, ed. 1982. *The Merck Manual of Diagnosis and Therapy*. Rahway, N.J.: Merck Sharp & Dohme Research Laboratories.

———. 1997. *The Merck Manual of Medical Information*. Whitehouse Station, N.J.: Merck Research Laboratories.

Berliner, Howard S. 1985. *A System of Scientific Medicine: Philanthropic Foundations in the Flexner Era*. New York: Tavistock Publications.

Bibel, D. J. 1988. *Milestones in Immunology: A Historical Exploration*. Madison: University of Wisconsin Press.

Black, Kathryn. 1996. *In the Shadow of Polio: A Personal and Social History*. Reading, Mass.: Addison-Wesley.

Blake, John B. 1948. The Origins of Public Health in the United States. *American Journal of Public Health* 38 (November): 1539–50.

Blancher, David. 1979. Workshops of the Revolution: A History of the Laboratories of the New York City Department of Health, 1892–1912. Ph.D. thesis, City University of New York.

Blank, Helen Lakin. 1983. The Responses of Physicians to Medical Reform: Health Care and the Medical Profession in New York City, 1890–1940. Ph.D. thesis, State University of New York, Stony Brook.

Blank, Robert H. 1993. *Fetal Protection in the Workplace: Women's Rights, Business Interests, and the Unborn*. New York: Columbia University Press.

Bloom, Charles James. 1919. Vaccine Therapy: The Most Rational and Effective Method of Treating Whooping Cough. *Archives of Pediatrics* 36: 1–27.

Blower, S. M., and A. R. McLean. 1994. Prophylactic Vaccines, Risk Behavior Change, and the Probability of Eradicating HIV in San Francisco. *Science* 265, no. 5177 (2 September): 1451–54.

Blumenthal, Ralph. 2007. Texas Is First to Require Cancer Shots for Schoolgirls. *The New York Times*, 3 February, p. A9.

Blumer, Herbert. 1969. Social Movements. In *Studies in Social Movements: A Social Psychological Perspective*, edited by Barry McLaughlin, 8–29. New York: The Free Press.

Bodewitz, J. H. W., Henk Buurma, and Gerard H. de Vries. 1987. Regulatory Science and the Social Management of Trust in Medicine. In *The Social Construction of Technological Systems: New Directions in the Sociology*

and History of Technology, edited by Wiebe B. Bijker, Thomas
P. Hughes, and Trevor J. Pinch, 243–59. Cambridge: MIT Press.

Bogert, Frank Vander. 1918. Experience with Vaccine in the Prevention of
Whooping Cough. *American Journal of Diseases of Children* 15: 271.

Bolognesi, Dani P. 1989. Progress in Vaccines against AIDS. *Science* 246,
no. 4935 (8 December): 1233–34.

Booth, William. 1987. Another Muzzle for AIDS Education? *Science* 238, no.
4830 (20 November): 1036.

———. 1988a. AIDS Policy in the Making. *Science* 239, no. 4844 (4 March):
1087.

———. 1988b. An Underground Drug for AIDS. *Science* 241, no. 4871
(9 September): 1279–81.

———. 1988c. No Longer Ignored, AIDS Funds Just Keep Growing. *Science*
242, no. 4880 (11 November): 858–59.

Bordet, J., and O. Gengou, 1906. Le Microbe de la Coqueluche. *Annales de
l'Institut Pasteur* 20: 731–41.

Boston Women's Health Book Collective. 1984. *Our Bodies, Ourselves*. New
York: Simon and Schuster.

Boué, André, Emile Papiernick-Berkhauer, and Sophie Lévy-Thierry. 1969.
Attenuated Rubella Virus in Women. *American Journal of Diseases of
Children* 118 (October): 230–33.

Brandt, Allan M. 1978. Polio, Politics, and Duplicity: Ethical Aspects in
the Development of the Salk Vaccine. *International Journal of Health
Sciences* 8: 257–70.

———. 1985. *No Magic Bullet: A Social History of Disease in the United States
since 1880*. New York: Oxford University Press.

———. 1988a. AIDS: From Social History to Social Policy. In *AIDS,
the Burdens of History*, edited by Elizabeth Fee and Daniel M. Fox, 147–71.
Berkeley: University of California Press.

———. 1988b. The Syphilis Epidemic and Its Relation to AIDS. *Science* 239, no.
4838 (22 January): 375–80.

Brody, M., and R. H. Sorley. 1947. Neurological Complications Following
Administration of Pertussis Vaccine. *New York State Medical Journal* 47:
1016–17.

Brown, E. Richard. 1979. *Rockefeller Medicine Men: Medicine and
Capitalism in America*. Berkeley: University of California Press.

Brown, Herbert R. 1912–13. The Immunizing Effect on Guinea-Pigs of Small
Doses of Diphtheria Toxin. *Journal of Medical Research* 27: 445–55.

Brunell, P. 1983. Impact of Litigation on Immunization in Children.
Pediatrics 82, no. 6: 822–23.

Brun-Vézinet, F., C. Rouzioux, L. Montagnier, S. Chamaret, J. Gruest, F. Barré-
Sinoussi, D. Geroldi, J. C. Chermann, J. McCormick, and S. Mitchell. 1984.
Prevalence of Antibodies to Lymphadenopathy-Associated Retrovirus in
African Patients with AIDS. *Science* 226, no. 4673 (26 October): 453–56.

Buckley, William F., Jr. 1986. Identify All the Carriers. *The New York Times*, 18 March, p. A27.

Burstein, Paul, Rachel L. Einwohner, and Jocelyn A Hollander. 1995. The Success of Political Movements: A Bargaining Perspective. In *The Politics of Social Protest: Comparative Perspectives on States and Social Movements*, edited by J. Craig Jenkins and Bert Klandermans, 275–95. Minneapolis: University of Minnesota Press.

Burton, Mike. 1986. AIDS and Female Circumcision. *Science* 231, no. 4743 (14 March): 1236.

Byard, Dever S. 1921. The Schick Test and Active Immunization with Toxin-Antitoxin in Private Practice. *Archives of Pediatrics* 38: 22–31.

Byers, R. K., and F. C. Moll. 1948. Encephalopathies Following Prophylactic Pertussis Vaccine. *Pediatrics* 1: 437–57.

Bynum, W. F., Stephen Lock, and Roy Porter, eds. 1992. *Medical Journals and Medical Knowledge: Historical Essays*. New York: Routledge, Chapman, & Hall.

Byrne, Earl B., J. M. Ryan, M. F. Randolph, and D. M. Horstmann. 1969. Live Attenuated Rubella Virus in Young Adult Women: Trials of Cendehill and HPV77DE5+IgG. *American Journal of Diseases of Children* 118: 234–36.

Byrne, Gregory. 1988. Panel Laments "Disarray" in Public Health System. *Science* 241, no. 4873 (23 September): 1591.

Calhoun, Craig, ed. 1992. Introduction: Habermas and the Public Sphere. In *Habermas and the Public Sphere*. Cambridge: MIT Press.

Campbell, Alastair V. 1975. Ethical Codes. In *Moral Dilemmas in Medicine: A Coursebook on Ethics for Doctors and Nurses, Appendix*. Edinburgh: Churchill Livingstone.

Carter, Richard. 1966. *Breakthrough: The Saga of Jonas Salk*. New York: Trident Press.

CCGHVE, *see* Coordinating Committee of the Global HIV/AIDS Vaccine Enterprise.

CDC, *see* Centers for Disease Control.

CDCP, *see* Centers for Disease Control and Prevention.

Centers for Disease Control. 1981. Pneumocystis Pneumonia—Los Angeles. *Morbidity and Mortality Weekly Report* 30 (5 June): 250–52.

———. 1984. Declining Rates of Rectal and Pharyngeal Gonorrhea among Males—New York City. *Morbidity and Mortality Weekly Report* 33: 295–97.

———. 1999. Nation Reports New Highs in Childhood Immunization Levels. CDC Press Release, 24 September (search CSC web site at *www.cdc.gov*).

———. 2000. Compressed Mortality for Pertussis. CDC WONDER/PC Data File, generated 7 October, 22:51.

———. 2003. More U.S. Children Are Getting Their Shots. CDC Press Release, 31 July (*cdc.gov/od/oc/media/pressrel/r030731.htm*).

——. 2006. *Epidemiology and Prevention of Vaccine-Preventable Diseases.* Washington, D.C.: Department of Health and Human Services.

Centers for Disease Control and Prevention. 1983. General Recommendations on Immunization. *MMWR* 32, no. 1 (14 January): 1–8, 13–17.

——. 2002. General Recommendations on Immunization: Recommendations of the Advisory Committee on Immunization Practices and the American Academy of Family Physicians. *MMWR* 51, no. RR-2 (8 February): 1–35.

——. 2004a. Flu Prevention 2004–2005: An Update (*fda.gov/fdac/ features/2004/604_flu.html*).

——. 2004b. Interim Influenza Vaccination Recommendations: 2004–05 (*hhs. gov/news/press/2004pres/20041005b.html*).

——. 2005. Seasonal Flu (*www.cdc.gov/flu/weekly/weeklyarchives2004-2005/ 04-05summary.htm*).

Chaitow, Leon. 1987. *Vaccination and Immunisation: Dangers, Delusions, and Alternatives (What Every Parent Should Know).* Somerset, N.J.: Saffron Walden.

Chase, Allan. 1982. *Magic Shots: A Human and Scientific Account of the Long and Continuing Struggle to Eradicate Infectious Diseases by Vaccination.* New York: William Morrow and Company.

Chaves, Sandra S., P. Gargiullo, J. X. Zhang, R. Civen, D. Guris, L. Mascola, and J. F. Seward. 2007. Loss of Vaccine-Induced Immunity to Varicella over Time. *New England Journal of Medicine* 356, no. 11 (15 March): 1121–29.

Cherry, J. D., P. A. Brunnell, G. S. Golden, and D. T. Karezon. 1988. Report of the Task Force on Pertussis and Pertussis Immunization. *Pediatrics* 81 (suppl.): 939–84.

Christakis, Nicholas A. 1988. The Ethical Design of an AIDS Vaccine Trial in Africa. *Hastings Center Report* 18, no. 3: 31–37.

Cockburn, Charles W. 1969. World Aspects of the Epidemiology of Rubella. *American Journal of Diseases of Children* 118: 115.

Cohen, Hans. 1978. Vaccination against Pertussis, Yes or No? In *International Symposium on Pertussis*, edited by Charles R. Manclark and James C. Hill. National Institutes of Health, DHEW: 79–1830.

Cohen, Jon. 1991a. AIDS Vaccine Meeting: International Trials Soon. *Science* 254, no. 5032 (1 November): 647.

——. 1991b. FDA Committee Raises AIDS Vaccine Hurdles. *Science* 254, no. 5035 (22 November): 1105.

——. 1992a. French Agency Exonerates Zagury. *Science* 255, no. 5042 (17 January): 280.

——. 1992b. Did Political Clout Win Vaccine Trial for MicroGeneSys? *Science* 258, no. 5080 (9 October): 211.

——. 1992c. MicroGeneSys Vaccine Trial Gets a Public Peer Review. *Science* 258, no. 5085 (13 November): 1079–80.

——. 1992d. Pediatric AIDS Vaccine Trials Set. *Science* 258, no. 5088 (4 December): 1568–70.

————. 1992e. NIH Panel OK's Vaccine Test—In a New Form. *Science* 258, no. 5088 (4 December): 1569.

————. 1992f. AIDS Vaccines: Trials Set in High-risk Populations. *Science* 258, no. 5089 (11 December): 1729.

————. 1992g. AIDS Vaccine: Is Older Better? *Science* 258, no. 5090 (18 December): 1880–81.

————. 1993a. MicroGeneSys: Peer Review Triumphs Over Lobbying. *Science* 262, no. 5146 (28 January): 463.

————. 1993b. Agencies Spar over Vaccine Trial. *Science* 259, no. 5096 (5 February): 752–53.

————. 1993c. A "Manhattan Project" for AIDS? *Science* 259, no. 5098 (19 February): 1112–14.

————. 1993d. MicroGeneSys: NIH Faces Down DOD. *Science* 260, no. 5106 (16 April): 288.

————. 1993e. What Are the Correlates of Protection? *Science* 260, no. 5112 (28 May): 1259.

————. 1993f. Jitters Jeopardize AIDS Vaccine Trials. *Science* 262, no. 5136 (12 November): 980–81.

————. 1993g. AIDS Vaccine Research: A New Goal: Preventing Disease, Not Infection. *Science* 262, no. 5141 (17 December): 1820–21.

————. 1994a. AIDS Vaccines: Are Researchers Racing Toward Success, or Crawling? *Science* 265, no. 5177 (2 September): 1373–75.

————. 1994b. Behavioral Conundrums. *Science* 264, no. 5162 (20 May): 1073.

————. 1994c. AIDS Vaccine Research: U.S. Panel Votes to Delay Real-World Vaccine Trials. *Science* 264, no. 5167 (24 June): 1839.

————. 1995 Searching for the Ideal Cohort. *Science* 270, no. 5238 (10 November): 905.

————. 1996. Results on News AIDS Drug Bring Cautious Optimism. *Science* 271, no. 5250 (9 January): 755–56.

————. 2001. *Shots in the Dark: The Wayward Search for an AIDS Vaccine.* New York: W. W. Norton.

Colebrook, L. 1954. *Wright, Provocative Doctor and Thinker.* London: Heineman.

Colgrove, James. 2002. The McKeown Thesis: A Historical Controversy and Its Enduring Influence. *American Journal of Public Health* 92, no. 5 (May): 725–29.

————. 2004. Between Persuasion and Compulsion: Smallpox Control in Brooklyn and New York, 1894–1902. *Bulletin of the History of Medicine* 78, no. 2: 349–78.

————. 2006. *State of Immunity: The Politics of Vaccination in Twentieth-Century America.* Berkeley: University of California Press.

Collier, James Lincoln. 2004. *Vaccines.* Tarrytown, N.Y.: Benchmark Books.

Connolly, Maureen. 2000. Are Vaccines Still Safe? *Ladies Home Journal* 117, no. 7 (July): 82.

Cooper, Louis Z., J. P. Giles, and Saul Krugman. 1968. Clinical Trial of Live

Attenuated Rubella Virus Vaccine, PRV-77 Strain. *American Journal of Diseases of Children* 115 (June): 656.

Cooper, Louis Z., Philip R. Ziring, Helene J. Weiss, B. A. Matters, and S. Krugman. 1969. Transient Arthritis after Rubella Vaccination. *American Journal of Diseases of Children* 118: 218–25.

Coordinating Committee of the Global HIV/AIDS Vaccine Enterprise. 2005. The Global HIV/AIDS Vaccine Enterprise: Scientific Strategic Plan. *PLoS Med* 2, no. 2: e25.

Cope, Z. 1966. *Almoth Wright, Founder of Modern Vaccine-Therapy.* London: Heineman.

Corea, Gena. 1985. *The Hidden Malpractice: How American Medicine Mistreats Women,* updated ed. New York: Harper Colphon.

Coulter, Harris, and Barbara Loe Fisher. 1991. *A Shot in the Dark: Why the "P" in the DPT May Be Hazardous to Your Child's Health.* Garden City Park, N.Y.: Avery Publishing Group.

Council on Pharmacy and Chemistry, American Medical Association. 1931. Pertussis Vaccine Omitted from N. N. R. *JAMA* 96, no. 8 (21 February): 613.

CPC, *see* Council on Pharmacy and Chemistry, American Medical Association.

Crain, Robert L., Elihu Katz, and Donald B. Rosenthal. 1969. *The Politics of Community Conflict: The Fluoridation Decision.* New York: Bobbs-Merrill.

Crocker, Ruth. 1998. Unsettling Perspectives: The Settlement Movement, the Rhetoric of Social History, and the Search for Synthesis. In *Contesting the Master Narrative: Essays in Social History,* edited by Jeffrey Cox and Shelton Stromquist, 175–209. Iowa City: University of Iowa Press.

Culliton, Barbara J. 1984. Five Firms with the Right Stuff. *Science* 225, no. 4667 (14 September): 1129.

———. 1990. Gallo Reports Mystery Break-In. *Science* 250, no. 4980 (26 October): 502.

Culotta, Elizabeth. 1991. Forecasting the Global AIDS Epidemic. *Science* 253, no. 5022 (23 August): 852–54.

Curran, J. W., W. M. Morgan, A. M. Hardy, H. W. Jaffe, W. W. Darrow, and W. R. Dowdle. 1985. The Epidemiology of AIDS: Current Status and Future Prospects. *Science* 229, no. 4720 (27 September): 1352–57.

Daitz, Ben. 2006. Vaccine Prevents Cervical Cancer. So, What's the Downside? *The New York Times,* May 23, p. F5.

Daniel, M. D., F. Kirchoff, S. C. Czajak, P. K. Sehgal, and R. C. Desrosiers. 1992. Protective Effects of a Live Attenuated SIV Vaccine with a Deletion in the nef Gene. *Science* 258, no. 5090 (18 December): 1938–41.

Daniel, M. D., N. L. Letvin, N. W. King, M. Kannagi, P. K. Sehgal, R. D. Hunt, P. J. Kanki, M. Essex, and R. C. Desrosiers. 1985. Isolation of T-Cell Tropic HTLV-III-Like Retrovirus from Macaques. *Science* 228, no. 4704 (7 June): 1201–4.

Daniels, Cynthia R. 1993. *At Women's Expense: State Power and the Politics of Fetal Rights*. Cambridge: Harvard University Press.

Davis, Mike. 2005. *The Monsters at Our Door*. New York: The New Press.

Davis, R. L., E. Marcuse, S. Black, H. Sheinfeld, B. Givens, J. Schwalbe, P. Ray, R. S. Thomas, and R. Chen. 1997. MMR3 Immunization at 4 to 5 Years and 10 to 12 Years of Age: A Comparison of Adverse Clinical Events After Immunization in the Vaccine Safety Datalink Project. *Pediatrics* 100, no. 5 (November): 891–92.

Deardorff, William H. 1908. A Preliminary Report of the Treatment of Pertussis with Diphtheritic Serum. *American Medicine* 3: 73–74.

della Porta, Donatella. 1999. Protest, Protesters, and Protest Policing: Public Discourses in Italy and Germany from the 1960s to the 1980s. In *How Social Movements Matter*, edited by Marco Giugni, Doug McAdam, and Charles Tilly, 66–96. Minneapolis: University of Minnesota Press.

Densmore, Emmet. 1982. *How Nature Cures, Comprising a New System of Hygiene*. New York: Stillman & Co.

Detels, R., J. T. Grayston, K. S. W. Kim, K. P. Chen, J. L. Gale, R. P. Beasley, and L. Gutman. 1969. Prevention of Clinical and Subclinical Rubella Infection. *American Journal of Diseases of Children* 118: 295.

Dorozynski, Alexander. 1991. French AIDS Researcher Cleared. *Science* 252, no. 5003 (12 April): 203.

Dorozynski, Alexander, and Alun Anderson. 1991. Deaths in Vaccine Trial Trigger French Inquiry. *Science* 252, no. 5005 (26 April): 501–2.

Dowling, Harry F. 1977. *Fighting Infection: Conquests of the Twentieth Century*. Cambridge, Mass.: Harvard University Press.

Drane, James F. 1985. The Many Faces of Competency. *Hastings Center Report* 15, no. 2 (April): 17–21.

Dudgeon, Alastair J. 1986. A Global View of Immunization Tactics and Strategies for the Control of Rubella. In *Vaccinating against Brain Syndromes: The Campaign against Measles and Rubella*, edited by Enest M. Gruenberg, 140–57. New York: Oxford University Press.

———. 1969. Congenital Rubella: Pathogenesis and Immunology. *American Journal of Diseases of Children* 118: 42.

Dudgeon, Alastair J., W. C. Marshall, and C. S. Peckham. 1969. Rubella Vaccine Trials in Adults and Children: Comparison of Three Attenuated Vaccines. *American Journal of Diseases of Children* 118: 234–36.

Duffy, John. 1974. *A History of Public Health in New York City: 1866–1966*. New York: Russel Sage.

———. 1990. *The Sanitarians: A History of American Public Health*. Urbana: University of Illinois Press.

Dunne, John. 1995. Drug and Vaccine Trials: Scientific, Ethical, and Legal Considerations. In *HIV Law, Ethics, and Human Rights: Text and Materials*, edited by Dayanth C. Jayasuriya, 202–34. New Delhi: United Nations Development Program Regional Project on HIV and Development.

Dunwoody, Sharon. 1986. *The Science Writing Inner Club: A Communication Link Between Science and the Lay Public*. New York: The Free Press.

Dye, Thomas. 1972. *Understanding Public Policy*. Englewood Cliffs, N.J.: Prentice Hall.

Eaton, Monroe D. 1949. Some Advances in Chemotherapy. *The Scientific Monthly* 68, no. 6: 373–85.

Edwards, Audrey. 2006. Mumps Watch: Parents Are Urged to Verify Child Immunization as Outbreak Spreads. *The Washington Post*, May 9, p. F1.

Ehrenreich, Barbara, and Dierdre English. 1979. *For Her Own Good: 150 Years of the Experts' Advice to Women*. Garden City, N.Y.: Anchor Books.

Ekunwe, Ebun O., and Ross Kessel. 1984. "Case Studies": Informed Consent in the Developing World. *Hastings Center Report* 14, no. 3 (June): 22–24.

Ellis, Janice Rider, and Elizabeth Ann Nowlis. 1994. *Nursing: A Human Needs Approach*. Philadelphia: J. B. Lippincott Company.

Emminghaus, H. 1870. Uber rubeolen. *Jahrbuch für Kinderheilkunde* 4: 47–59. Cited in John J. Witte, A. W. Karchmer, G. Case, K. L. Herrmann, E. Abrutyn , I. Kassanoff, and J. S. Neill. Epidemiology of Rubella. *American Journal of Diseases of Children* 118: 107–11.

EPI, *see* Expanded Programme on Immunization.

Epstein, Steven. 1996. *Impure Science: AIDS, Activism and the Politics of Knowledge*. Berkeley: University of California Press.

Erhardt, Carl L. 1974. *Mortality and Morbidity in the United States*. Cambridge: Harvard University Press.

Ewick, Patricia, and Susan Silbey. 2003. *Narrating Social Structure: Stories of Resistance to Legal Authority. American Journal of Sociology* 108, no. 6 (May): 1328–72.

Expanded Programme on Immunization. 1991. Rubella and Congenital Rubella Syndrome in Developing Countries. WHO Document EPI/GAG/91/WP.15.

Faigman, David L. 2004. *Laboratory of Justice*. New York: Times Books.

Farquar, John D., and Jorge E. Corretjer. 1969. Clinical Experience with Cendehill Rubella Vaccine in Mature Women. *American Journal of Diseases of Children* 118: 326–28.

Fee, Elizabeth. 2000. The Rise and Fall of Public Health in the Twentieth Century. Paper presented in the Burroughs-Wellcome Public Health Series at the New York Academy of Medicine, 7 February.

Fee, Elizabeth, and Evelynn M. Hammonds. 1995. Science, Politics, and the Art of Persuasion: Promoting the New Scientific Medicine in New York City. In *Hives of Sickness*, edited by David Rosner, 155–96. New Brunswick, N.J.: Rutgers University Press.

Feldman, Eric. 1985. Medical Ethics the Japanese Way. *Hastings Center Report* 15, no. 5 (October): 21–24.

Felton, Harriet M., and Cynthia Y. Willard. 1944. Current Status of Prophylaxis by Hemophilus Pertussis. *JAMA* 126, no. 5 (September 30): 294–99.

Fenishel, G. M. 1983. The Pertussis Vaccine Controversy: The Danger of Case Reports. *Archives of Neurology* 40: 193–94.

Fenner, Frank. 1989. *Smallpox and Its Eradication*. Geneva: World Health Organization.

Fine, Ralph. 1972. *The Great Drug Deception*. New York: Stein & Day.

Finnegan, Francis A. 1920. Institutional Control of Diphtheria. *Boston Medical and Surgical Journal* 182: 93–94.

Fisher, Barbara Loe. 2000. Personal communication to the author, 18 July.

Fleck, L. 1979. *The Genesis and Development of a Scientific Fact*. Chicago: University of Chicago Press.

Flynn, N. M., D. N. Forthal, C. D. Harro, F. N. Judson, K. H. Mayer, and M. F. Para. 2005. Placebo-Controlled Phase 3 Trial of a Recombinant Glycoprotein 120 Vaccine to Prevent HIV-1 Infection. *The Journal of Infectious Diseases* 191, no. 5 (1 March): 654–65.

Forbes, John A. 1969. Rubella: Historical Aspects. *American Journal of Diseases of Children* 118: 5.

Fox, Max J., and Mortimer M. Bortin. 1952. Rubella in Pregnancy Causing Malformation in Newborn. *JAMA* 130: 132–33.

Francis, Donald P., and James Chin. 1987. The Prevention of Acquired Immunodeficiency Syndrome in the United States: An Objective Strategy for Medicine, Public Health, Business, and the Community. *JAMA* 257, no. 10 (13 March): 1357–66.

Franklin, D. 1984. Rubella Threatens Unborn in Vaccine Gap. *Science News* 125 (24 March): 186.

Freed, Gary L., W. Clayton Bordley, and Gordon H. Defriese. 1993. Childhood Immunization Programs: An Analysis of Policy Issues. *The Milbank Quarterly* 71, no. 1: 65–96.

Frenkel, L. D., and K. Nielsen. 2003. Immunization Issues for the 21st Century. *Annals of Allergy, Asthma & Immunology* 90, no. 6 (June Supp. 3): 45–52.

Freudenheim, Milt. 2007. Showdown Looms in Congress Over Drug Advertising on TV. *The New York Times*, 22 January, p. C1.

Friedan, Betty. 1963. *The Feminine Mystique*. New York: W. W. Norton.

Friedson, Eliot. 1973. *The Profession of Medicine*. New York: Dodd, Mead, and Company.

Fukuda, Keiji. 2005. U.S. Influenza Surveillance 2004–2005 *(www.fda.gov/ohrms/dockets/ac/05/slides/2005-4087S1_2.pdf)*.

Fulginiti, Vincent A. 1983. Letter to the Editor. *American Journal of Diseases in Children* 137 (September): 923.

———. 1992. How Safe Are Pertussis and Rubella Vaccines? A Commentary on the Institute of Medicine Report. *Pediatrics* 89, no. 2: 334–36.

Fuller, R., and R. Myers. 1941. The Natural History of a Social Problem. *American Sociological Review* 6, no. 3: 320–29.

Furman, Bess. 1955. One Firm's Vaccine Barred; 6 Polio Cases Studied. *New York Times*, 28 April, p. 1ff.

Gabe, Jonathan, ed. 1995. *Medicine, Health, and Risk: Sociological Approaches*. Oxford: Blackwell Publishing.

Galambos, Louis, and Jane Eliot Sewell. 1995. *Networks of Innovation: Vaccine Development at Merck Sharp & Dohme, and Mulford: 1895–1995.* Cambridge: Cambridge University Press.

Gallo, Robert C., Prem S. Sarin, E. P. Gelmann, M. Robert-Guroff, E. Richardson, V. S. Kalyanaraman, D. Mann, G. D. Sidhu, R. E. Stahl, S. Zolla-Pazner, J. Leibowitch, and M. Popovic. 1983. Isolation of Human T-Cell Leukemia Virus in Acquired Immune Deficiency Syndrome (AIDS). *Science* 220, no. 4599 (20 May): 865–67.

Gallo, Robert C., S. Z. Salahuddin, M. Popovic, G. M. Shearer, M. Kaplan, B. F. Haynes, T. J. Palker, R. Redfield, J. Oleske, B. Safai. 1984. Frequent Detection and Isolation of Cytopathic Retroviruses (HTLV-III) from Patients with AIDS and at Risk for AIDS. *Science* 224 (4 May): 500–502.

Gamble, S. W. 1986. AIDS: Responding to the Crisis; a Public Policy Agenda. *Health Progress* 67, no. 4 (May): 30–33.

Gamble, V. N. 1991. Under the Shadow of Tuskegee: African Americans and Health Care. *American Journal of Public Health* 87: 1773–78.

GCCSE, *see* Global Commission for the Certification of Smallpox Eradication.

Gerth, H. H., and C. Wright Mills. 1978. *From Max Weber: Essays in Sociology.* New York: Oxford University Press.

Global Commission for the Certification of Smallpox Eradication. 1980. *The Global Eradication of Smallpox.* Geneva: World Health Organization.

Globus, J. H. and J. L. Kohn. 1949. Encephalopathy Following Pertussis Vaccine Prophylaxis. *JAMA* 141: 507.

Gold, Jerome A., Abel Prinzie, and James McKee. 1969. Adult Women Vaccinated with Rubella Vaccine: A Preliminary Report on Controlled Studies with Cendehill Strain. *American Journal of Diseases of Children* 118: 264–65.

Goldsmith, M. F. 1991. Can't Find One AIDS Vaccine? Try for a Few! *JAMA* 266, no. 6 (14 August): 763–64.

Goldstein, Martin, and Inge F. Goldstein. 1980. *How We Know: An Exploration of the Scientific Process.* New York: Da Capo Press.

Goler, George W. 1917. Whooping cough is prevented by vaccination. *New York State Journal of Medicine* 17: 411–13.

González, Elizabeth Rasche. 1982. TV Report on DPT Galvanizes U. S. Pediatricians. *JAMA* 248, no. 1: 12–23.

Goodman, Herbert M. 1908. The Duration and Disappearance of Passive Diphtheric Immunity. *Journal of Infectious Disease* 15: 153, 181–84.

Gostin, L. O. 1989. Public Health Strategies for Confronting AIDS: Legislative and Regulatory Policy in the United States. *JAMA* 261, no. 11: 1621–30.

Goubert, J. P. 1987. Twenty Years On: Problems of Historical Methodology in the History of Health. In *Problems and Methods in the History of Medicine*, edited by Roy Porter and Andrew Wear, 40–56. London: Croom Helm.

Grady, Denise. 2006a. Doubt Cast on Stockpile of a Vaccine for Bird Flu. *The New York Times*, 30 March, p. A20.

———. 2006b. The Vaccine, It Seems, Lacks Moxie. *The New York Times*, 23 April, p. 42.

Graham, Edwin E. 1911. The Treatment of Pertussis with Vaccine. *Transactions of the American Pediatric Society* 23: 157–66.

Grandy, C. R. 1909. Whooping Cough from the Point of View of Public Health. *JAMA* 52 2094–96.

Green, Robert H., Michael R. Balsamo, Joan P. Giles, Saul Krugman, and George Mirick. 1965. Studies on the Natural History and Prevention of Rubella. *American Journal of Diseases of Children* 110: 348–65.

Greenberg, Morris, Ottavio Pellitteri, and Jerome Barton. 1957. Frequency of Defects in Infants Whose Mothers Had Rubella During Pregnancy. *JAMA* 185, no. 6 (12 October): 675–78.

Gregg, N. M. 1941. Congenital Cataract Following German Measles in the Mother. *Transactions of the Ophthalmological Society of Australia* 3, no. 33: 46.

Gruenberg, Ernest M., Carol Lewis, and Stephen E. Goldston. 1986. *Vaccinating against Brain Syndromes: The Campaign against Measles and Rubella*. New York: Oxford University Press.

Gust, Deborah A., Tara W. Strine, Emmanuel Maurice, Philip Smith, Hussain Yusuf, Marilyn Wilkinson, Michael Battaglia, Robert Wright, and Benjamin Schwartz. 2004. Underimmunization Among Children: Effects of Vaccine Safety Concerns on Immunization Status. *Pediatrics* 114: e16–e22.

Guthrie, Hilda Jeanette. 1977. Differences in the Characteristics and Opinions of Those Persons Taking and Those Persons Not Taking the Swine Flu Vaccine in East Tennessee. Ph.D. thesis, University of Tennessee.

Haller, John S. 1994. *Medical Protestants: The Eclectics in American Medicine*. Carbondale: Southern Illinois University Press.

Halpern, Sydney. 2004. *Lesser Harms: The Morality of Risk in Medical Research*. Chicago: University of Chicago Press.

Hammonds, Evelynn M. 1993. The Search for Perfect Control: A Social History of Diphtheria. Ph.D. thesis, Harvard University.

———. 1999. *Childhood's Deadly Scourge: The Campaign to Control Diphtheria in New York City, 1880–1930*. Baltimore: The Johns Hopkins University Press.

Hansen, Bert. 1998. America's First Medical Breakthrough: How Popular Excitement about a French Rabies Cure Raised New Expectations for Medical Progress. *American Historical Review* 103, no. 2: 373–418.

Hardy, Anne. 1993. *The Epidemic Streets: Infectious Disease and the Rise of Preventive Medicine, 1856–1900*. Oxford: Clarendon Press.

Harris, Gardiner. 2006. Vaccine against Diarrhea-Causing Virus Is Approved. *The New York Times*, 4 February.

Hart, Lianne. 2007. Uproar over HPV Vaccine Order. *The Los Angeles Times* (25 February), p. A25.

Hartshorn, W. Morgan, and Henry Nicholas Moeller. 1914. Vaccine Treatment in Pertussis. *Archives of Pediatrics* 31: 586–98.

Haseltine, W. A., and J. A. Levy. 1991. HIV Research and *nef* Alleles. *Science* 253, no. 5018 (26 July): 366.

Hefernan, Roy J., and William A. Lynch. 1953. What is the Status of Therapeutic Abortion in Modern Obstetrics? *American Journal of Obstetrics and Gynecology* 66, no. 2: 335.

Heinemann, P. G., and A. C. Hicks. 1909. Bleeding to Death in Order to Obtain Maximum Amount of Anti-diphtheric Serum from Horses. *Journal of Infectious Disease* 6: 615–18.

Heller, Jacob. 2000. Rubella Vaccine and Medical Policy-Making: Fetal Rights and Women's Health. *New England Journal of Public Policy* 16, no. 1 (fall/winter): 117–38.

———. 2005. Mobilizing against Vaccination Mandates: The Case of NY Assembly Bill 9988-A. *National Social Science Journal* 25, no. 1: 77–84.

Henderson, D. A. 1987. Principles and Lessons from the Smallpox Eradication Programme. *Bulletin of the World Health Organization* 65: 535–46.

Henican, Ellis. 2007. Why a Lifesaving Shot Isn't Yet Mandatory. *Newsday*, 12 January, p. A2.

Hess, A. F. 1914. The Use of a Series of Vaccines in the Prophylaxis and Treatment of an Epidemic of Pertussis. *American Journal of Obstetrics* 69, 510–12.

Hill, Bradford A., and T. M. Galloway. 1949. Maternal Rubella and Congenital Defects: Data From National Health Insurance Records. *Lancet* 1: 299.

Hilleman, M. R. 1992. Past, Present, and Future of Measles, Mumps, and Rubella Virus Vaccines. *Pediatrics* 90, no. 1: 149–53.

Hinman, A. R., H. Foege, C. A. de Quartos, P. A. Patriarca, W. A. Orenstein, and E. W. Brink. 1987. The Case for Global Eradication of Poliomyelitis. *Bulletin of the World Health Organization* 67: 835–40.

Hoeckelman, Robert A. 1997. *Primary Pediatric Care*, 3d ed. St. Louis: Mosby.

Hoffman, Lily. 1989. *The Politics of Knowledge: Activist Movements in Medicine and Planning*. Albany, N.Y.: SUNY Press.

Hofstadter, Richard. 1964. *The Paranoid Style in American Politics and Other Essays*. New York: Vintage Books.

———. 1966. *Anti-Intellectualism in American Life*. New York: Vintage Books.

Holden, Constance. 1992. Zagury in the Clear. *Science* 255, no. 5045 (7 February): 680.

———. 1993. Zagury Probe Concluded. *Science* 260, no. 5109 (7 May): 757.

———. 1994. Weighing HIV Vaccine Trials. *Science* 265, no. 5173 (5 August): 735.

———. 1995. Education Booster for AIDS. *Science* 268, no. 5207 (7 April): 35.

Hollingsworth, J. Rogers, Jerald Hage, and Robert A. Hanneman. 1990. *State*

Intervention in Medical Care: Consequences for Britain, France, Sweden, and the United States. Ithaca, N.Y.: Cornell University Press.

———. 1986. *A Political Economy of Medicine: Great Britain and the United States.* Baltimore: The Johns Hopkins Press.

Horstmann, Dorothy M., J. E. Banatvala, J. T. Riordan, M. C. Payne, R. Whittimore, E. M. Opton, and C. du Ve Florey. 1965. Rubella Symposium. *American Journal of Diseases of Children* 110 (October): 409.

Howson, Christopher P., and Harvey V. Fineberg. 1992a. Adverse Effects Following Pertussis and Rubella Vaccines: Summary of a Report of the Institute of Medicine. *JAMA* 267, no. 3 (15 January): 392–96.

———. 1992b. The Ricochet of Magic Bullets: Summary of the Institute of Medicine Report, *Adverse Effects of Pertussis and Rubella Vaccines.* Pediatrics 189, no. 2: 318–24.

Howson, Christopher P., Cynthia J. Howe, and Harvey V. Fineberg, eds. 1991. *Adverse Effects of Pertussis and Rubella Vaccines.* Washington, D. C.: National Academy Press.

Howson, Christopher P., M. Katz, R. B. Johnston, Jr., and H. V. Fineberg. 1992. Chronic Arthritis After Rubella Vaccination. *Clinical Infectious Diseases* 15, no. 2: 307–12.

Huenekens, E. J. 1917. The Prophylactic Use of Pertussis Vaccine Controlled by the Complement Fixation Test. *American Journal of Diseases of Children* 14: 283–86.

———. 1918. Further Report on the Use of Pertussis Vaccine Controlled by the Complement Fixation Test. *American Journal of Diseases of Children* 16: 30–33.

Hughes, S. S. 1977. *The Virus: A History of the Concept.* New York: Heinemann Educational Books.

Hutchins, Sarah Ann, and Risa Eckes. 1994. Clinical Research: Considerations for Prospective Participants. *Nursing Clinics of North America* 31, no. 1: 25–35.

IAVI, *see* International AIDS Vaccine Initiative.

Imperato, Pascal James. 1974. *The Treatment and Control of Infectious Diseases in Man.* Springfield, Ill.: Charles Thomas.

———. 1983. *The Administration of a Public Health Agency: A Case Study of the New York City Department of Health.* New York: Human Sciences Press, Inc.

Inglhart, John K. 1987. Compensating Children with Vaccine-Related Injuries. *New England Journal of Medicine* 316, no. 20 (May): 1283–88.

Institute of Medicine. 1985. *Vaccine Supply and Innovation.* Washington, D.C.: National Academy Press.

———. 1986. *Confronting AIDS: Directions for Public Health, Health Care, and Research.* Washington, D.C.: National Academy Press.

———. 1988. *Confronting AIDS: Directions for Public Health, Health Care, and Research,* Update 1988 (Part I). Washington, D.C.: National Academy Press.

International AIDS Vaccine Initiative. 2004. Global Investment and Expenditures on Preventive HIV Vaccines: Methods and Results for 2002. *IAVI Policy Reseach Working Paper* (*www.iavi.org/file.cfm?fid=405*).

IOM, *see* Institute of Medicine.

Isaacson, Nicole. 1996. The "Fetus-Infant": Changing Classifications of *In Utero* Development in Medical Texts. *Sociological Forum* 11, no. 3: 457–80.

James, Frank. 2004. Flu Crisis Exposes Large Gaps in Bioterrorism Readiness; Experts: More Progress Needed. *Chicago Tribune*, 28 November, p. 14.

James, Walene. 1995. *Immunization: The Reality Behind the Myth*. Westport, Conn.: Bergin & Garvey.

Jardine, Nicholas. 1992. The Laboratory Revolution in Medicine as Rhetorical and Aesthetic Accomplishment. In *The Laboratory Revolution in Medicine*, edited by Andrew Cunningham and Perry Williams, 304–23. New York: Cambridge University Press.

Jasanoff, Sheila. 1997. *Science at the Bar*. Cambridge: Harvard University Press.

Jenner, Edward. 1938[1800]. Continuation of Facts and Observations Relative to the *Variolae Vaccinae*, or Cow-pox. In *The Harvard Classics*, Volume 38, 203–20. New York: P.F. Collier & Son.

Jenness, David. 1986. Scientists' Role in AIDS Control. *Science* 233, no. 4766 (22 August): 825.

Johnson, Judith A. 1998. *AIDS Funding for Federal Government Programs: FY1981-FY1999*. CRS Report for Congress. Washington, D.C.: Congressional Research Service (*http://opencrs.cdt.org/document/ Updated/1998–03-31%2000:00:00*).

Jones, James H. 1981. *Bad Blood: The Tuskegee Syphilis Experiment*. New York: Free Press.

———. 1992. The Tuskegee Legacy: AIDS and the Black Community. *Hastings Center Report* 22, no. 6 (November/December): 38–40.

Judson, F. N. 1983. Fear of AIDS and Gonorrhea Rates in Homosexual Men. *Lancet* 2, no. 8342 (16 July): 159–60.

Kaiser, Jocelyn. 1995. Chimp Finally Shows AIDS Symptoms. *Science* 270, no. 5234 (13 October): 223.

Kaplan, Temma. 1997. *Crazy for Democracy: Women in Grassroots Movements*. New York: Routledge.

Karzon, D. T. 1969. Panel Discussion on Future of Rubella Virus Vaccines. *American Journal of Diseases of Children* 118: 384.

Katz, Elihu, Martin L. Levin, and Herbert Hamilton. 1963. Traditions of Research on the Diffusion of Innovation. *American Sociological Review* 28, no. 2 (April): 237–52.

Katz, M. 1974. Rubella Vaccine. *The Journal of Pediatrics* 84, no. 4: 615–16.

Kaufman, Martin. 1967. The American Anti-Vaccinationists. *Bulletin of the History of Medicine* 41: 463–78.

Kendrick, Pearl. 1975. Can Whooping Cough Be Eradicated? *Journal of Infectious Disease* 132: 707–12.

Kendrick, Pearl, and G. Elderling. 1935. The Significance of Bacteriological

Methods in the Diagnosis and Control of Whooping Cough. *American Journal of Public Health* 25 (February): 147–55.

———. 1936. Progress Report of Pertussis Immunization. *American Journal of Public Health and the Nation's Health* 26 (January): 8–12.

———. 1939. A Study in Active Immunization against Pertussis. *American Journal of Hygiene* 29 (May): 133–53.

Kerns, Thomas A. 1997. *Ethical Issues in HIV Vaccine Trials*. New York: St Martin's Press.

King, Lester. 1991. *Transformations in American Medicine: From Benjamin Rush to William Osler*. Baltimore: Johns Hopkins University Press.

Kirp, David L., and Hugh Maher. 1987. The Politics of the AIDS Vaccine: Or How the California Legislature Searched for the Magic Bullet—and Wound Up Squabbling with the Trial Lawyers, the Budget Cutters, and the Alzheimer's Establishment, working paper, No. 87-7. Berkeley: Institute of Governmental Studies.

Klein, Aaron. 1972. *Trial by Fury*. New York: Doubleday.

Knoll, Elizabeth. 1992. The American Medical Association and Its Journal. In *Medical Journals and Medical Knowledge: Historical Essays*, edited by W.F. Bynum, Stephen Lock, and Roy Porter, 146–64. New York: Routledge, Chapman, & Hall.

Knorr-Cetina, Karin. 1981. *Manufacture of Knowledge: An Essay on the Constructivist and Contextual Nature of Science*. Oxford: Pergamon Press.

Koff, Wayne C. 1994. The Next Step Towards a Global AIDS Vaccine. *Science* 266, no. 5189 (25 November): 1335–37.

Koff, Wayne C., and Daniel F. Hoth. 1988. Development and Testing of AIDS Vaccines. *Science* 241, no. 4864 (22 July): 426–32.

Kohler, Robert E. 1979. Medical Reform and Biomedical Science. In *The Therapeutic Revolution*, edited by Morris Vogel and Charles E. Rosenberg. Philadelphia: University of Pennsylvania Press.

Kolata, Gina. 1983. Congress, NIH Open Coffers for AIDS: Fear, Political Pressure, and Scientific Interest Have Prompted a Surge of Research Funds; the Course of the Epidemic Remains Hard to Predict. *Science* 221, no. 4609 (29 July): 436–38.

Kraut, Alan. 1994. *Silent Travelers: Germs, Genes, and the Immigrant Menace*. New York: Basic Books.

Kriesi, Hanspeter. The Organizational Structure of New Social Movements in a Political Context. In *Comparative Perspectives on Social Movements*, edited by Doug McAdam, John D. McCarthy, and Mayer Zald, 153–84. New York: Cambridge University Press.

Krim, Mathilde. 1985. AIDS: The Challenge to Science and Medicine. *Hastings Center Report* 15, no. 4 (August): 2–7.

Krugman, Saul. 1969. Panel Discussion on Future of Rubella Virus. *American Journal of Diseases of Children* 118: 382.

Kuhn, Thomas. 1962. *The Structure of Scientific Revolutions.* Chicago: University of Chicago Press.

Kulenkampff, H., J. S. Schwartzman, and J. Wilson. 1974. Neurological Complications of Pertussis Inoculation. *Archives of Diseases in Children* 49: 46–49.

Kunz, Jeffrey R. M., ed. 1982. *The American Medical Association Family Medical Guide.* New York: Random House.

Kuttner, Robert. 2004. Bush Is Idle in Flu-Shot Fiasco. *Boston Globe,* 27 October, p. A19.

Ladd, Maynard. 1912. Vaccines in the Treatment of Pertussis. *Archives of Pediatrics* 29, 581–84.

Lancet. 1946. Medicine and the Law. *Lancet* 1: 208.

Lasky, L. A., J. E. Groopman, C. W. Fennie, P. M. Benz, D. J. Capon, D. J. Dowbenko, G. R. Nakamura, W. M. Nunes, M. E. Renz, and P. W. Berman. 1986. Neutralization of the AIDS Retrovirus by Antibodies to a Recombinant Envelope Glycoprotein. *Science* 233, no. 4760 (11 July): 209–12.

Latour, Bruno. 1987. *Science in Action.* Cambridge: Harvard University Press.

———. 1988. *The Pasteurization of France.* Cambridge: Harvard University Press.

Latour, Bruno, and Steven Woolgar. 1986. *Laboratory Life: The Construction of Scientific Facts.* Princeton: Princeton University Press.

Leary, Mark R., and Lisa S. Schreindorfer. 1998. The Stigmatization of HIV and AIDS. In *HIV & Social Interaction,* edited by Valerian J. Derlaga and Anita P. Barbee, 12–29. Thousand Oaks, Calif.: Sage Publications.

Leavitt, Judith Walzer. 1986. *Brought to Bed: Childbearing in America, 1750 to 1950.* New York: Oxford University Press.

———. 2003. Public Resistance or Cooperation? A Tale of Smallpox in Two Cities. *Biosecurity and Bioterrorism: Biodefense Strategy, Practice, and Science* 1, no. 3: 185–92.

Lee, Orville. 1999. Social Theory Across Disciplinary Boundaries: Cultural Studies and Sociology. *Sociological Forum* 14, no. 4: 547–81.

Lee, Ryan. 2005. Activists Raise Ethics Issues of HIV Prevention Trials. *Washington Blade* (10 June). Search *www.washblade.com/advancedsearch.*

Lee, Tun-Hou. 1997. Acquired Immunodeficiency Disease Vaccines: Design and Development. In *AIDS Etiology, Diagnosis, Treatment, and Prevention,* edited by Vincent T. Devita, Samuel Hellman, and Steven A. Rosenberg, 605–16. Philadelphia: Lippincott-Raven.

Leonard, J. M., J. W. Abramczuk, D. S. Pezen, R. Rutledge, J. H. Belcher, F. Hakim, G. Shearer, L. Lamperth, W. Travis, and T. Fredrickson. 1988. Development of Disease and Virus Recovery in Transgenic Mice Containing HIV Proviral DNA. *Science* 242, no. 4886 (23 December): 1665–70.

Lepow, Martha L., J. A. Veronelli, D. D. Hostetler, and F. C. Robbins. 1968. A Trial with Live Attenuated Rubella Vaccine. *American Journal of Diseases of Children* 115 (June): 639–47.

Levy, E. C. 1909. Annual Report of the Health Department of Richmond. In Grandy, C. R. 1909. Whooping Cough from the Point of View of Public Health. *JAMA* 52, 2094–96.

Lin, D. B., C. L. Kao, and C. Y. Lee. 1996. Study of Young Women Vaccinated against Rubella Virus for 10 Years in Taiwan. *Southeast Asian Journal of Tropical Medicine & Public Health* 27, no. 4 (December): 707–14.

Linders, Annulla. 1998. Moral Politics: Abortion and Capital Punishment Sweden and the United States, 1800–1980. Ph.D. thesis, State University of New York, Stony Brook.

Linke, Uli. 1986. AIDS in Africa. *Science* 231, no. 4735 (17 January): 203.

Logan, W. P. D. 1954. The Effects of Virus Infections in Pregnancy: A Historical Review of the Relationship of Congenital Effect and Rubella. *Medicine Illustrated* 8, no. 8: 502–4.

Long, Perrin H. 1949. Aureomycin. *The Scientific Monthly* 69, no. 1 (July): 3–8.

Löwy, Ilana. 1992. The Strength of Loose Concepts—Boundary Concepts, Federative Experimental Strategies and Disciplinary Growth: The Case of Immunology. *History of Science* 30: 371–96.

Luker, Kristin. 1984. *Abortion and the Politics of Motherhood.* Berkeley: University of California Press.

Luttinger, Paul. 1917. Pertussis Vaccine, Its Value as a Curative a Prophylactic Agent in Whooping Cough. *JAMA* 68, 1461–64.

Maayan-Metzger, A., P. Kedem-Friedrich, and J. Kuint. 2005. To Vaccinate or Not to Vaccinate—That Is the Question: Why Are Some Mothers Opposed to Giving Their Infants Hepatitis B Vaccine? *Vaccine* 23, no. 16 (March 14): 1941–48.

MacEvitt, James. 1910. Pertussis. *American Journal of Obstetrics* 61, 545–52.

Macklin, Ruth. 2004. *Double Standards in Medical Research in Developing Countries.* New York: Cambridge University Press.

MacLeod, R. M. 1967. Law, Medicine, and Public Opinion: The Resistance to Compulsory Health Legislation 1870–1907 (Parts I and II). *Public Law* (summer): 107–28, 189–211.

Madsen, Thorvald. 1925. Whooping Cough: Its Bacteriology, Diagnosis, Prevention, and Treatment. *Boston Medical and Surgical Journal* 192, no. 2: 50–60.

———. 1933. Vaccination against Whooping Cough. *JAMA* 101, no. 3 (15 July): 187–88.

Maines, David R. 1999. Information Pools and Racialized Narrative Structure. *The Sociological Quarterly* 40, no. 2: 317–20.

Malle, Louis. 1982. *My Dinner with Andre.* Fox Lorber.

Manclark, Charles R., and James C. Hill., eds. 1979. Discussion. In *International Symposium on Pertussis*, 311–15. Washington, D.C.: U.S. Department of Health, Education, and Welfare.

Manier, Jeremy. 2004. Flu Shot Eligibility Lowered to Age 50; Low Demand Eases National Shortage. *Chicago Tribune*, 18 December, p. 1.

Manton, W. G. 1815. Some Accounts of Rash Liable to be Mistaken for Scarlatina. *Medical Transactions of the Royal College of Physicians 5*, 149–65. Quoted in Preblud, Stephen R., Alan R. Hinman, and Kenneth L. Herrmann. 1980. An Evaluation of the United States' Rubella Immunization Program. *American Annals of the Deaf* 125: 968–76.

Marcuse, Edgar K. 1992. Obstacles to Immunization in the Public Sector. *25th National Immunization Conference Proceedings, June 10–14, 1991.* Washington, D.C.: U.S. Department of Health and Human Services (March): 87–90.

Mariner, Wendy K. 1989. Why Clinical Trials of AIDS Vaccines are Premature. *American Journal of Public Health* 79, no. 1 (January): 86–91.

Markowitz, G. E., and D. K. Rosner. 1973. Doctors in Crisis: A Study of the Use of Medical Education Reform to Establish Modern Professional Elitism in Medicine. *American Quarterly* 25: 83–107.

Marks, Harry M. 1997. *The Progress of Experiment: Science and Therapeutic Reform in the United States, 1900–1990.* New York: Cambridge University Press.

Marshall, Eliot. 1989. Quick Release of AIDS Drugs. *Science* 245, no. 4916 (28 July): 345–47.

Martin, Brian. 1989. The Sociology of the Fluoridation Controversy: A Reexamination. *The Sociological Quarterly* 30, no. 1: 59–76.

Martin, Emily. 1994. *Flexible Bodies: Tracking Immunity in American Culture —From the Days of Polio to the Age of AIDS.* Boston: Beacon Press.

Marx, Gary T., and Douglas McAdam. 1994. *Collective Behavior and Social Movements: Process and Structure.* Englewood Cliffs, N.J.: Prentice Hall.

Marx, Jean L. 1983. Human T-Cell Leukemia Virus Linked to AIDS. *Science* 220, no. 4599 (20 May): 806–9.

———. 1984. Strong New Candidate for AIDS Agent. *Science* 224, no. 4648 (4 May): 475–77.

———. 1985. A Virus by Any Other Name. *Science* 227, no. 4693 (22 March): 1449–51.

———. 1986. AIDS Virus Has New Name—Perhaps. *Science* 232, no. 4751 (9 May): 699–700.

———. 1987. The AIDS Virus—Well Known but a Mystery. *Science* 236, no. 4800 (24 April): 390–92.

———. 1989. AIDS Drugs—Coming but Not Here. *Science* 244, no. 4902 (21 April): 287.

Maulitz, Russell C. 1979. "Physician vs. Bacteriologist": The Ideology of Science in Clinical Medicine. In*The Therapeutic Revolution: Essays in the Social History of American Medicine,* edited by Morris J. Vogel and Charles E. Rosenberg, 91–107. Philadelphia: University of Pennsylvania Press.

Mazumdar, Pauline M. H. 1995. *Species and Specificity: An Interpretation of the History of Immunology.* New York: Cambridge University Press.

McCarthy, John, and Mayer Zald. *The Trend in Social Movements in*

America: Professionalization and Resource Mobilization. Morristown, N.J.: General Learning Press.

McCarthy, John D., Jackie Smith, and Mayer N. Zald. 1996. Accessing Public, Media, Electoral, and Governmental Agendas. In *Comparative Perspectives on Social Movements*, edited by Doug McAdam, John D. McCarthy, and Mayer Zald, 291–311. New York: Cambridge University Press.

McClintock, Charles T., and Newell S. Ferry. 1911. Production of Immunity with Over-Neutralized Diphtheria Toxin. *Zentralblatt für Bakteriologie 59*, 456–64.

McKenna, M. A. J. 2006. Vaccine to Avert Bird Flu Falls Short. *Atlanta Journal-Constitution*, 30 March, p. B1.

McKeown, Thomas. 1976. *The Modern Rise of Population*. London: Edward Arnold.

McKinlay John B., and Sonja M. McKinlay. 1977. The Questionable Contributions of Medical Measures to the Decline of Mortality in the United States in the Twentieth Century. *Milbank Memorial Fund Quarterly/Health and Society 55*, no. 3: 405–28.

McLeod, R. M. 1967. Law, Medicine and Public Opinion: The Resistance to Compulsory Health Legislation 1870–1907, Parts I and II. *Public Law*: 107–28, 189–211.

McNeil, Donald R. 1985. America's Longest War: The Fight over Fluoridation, 1950–. *The Wilson Quarterly 9*, no. 3 (Summer): 140–53.

Meckel, Richard A. 1990. *Save the Babies: American Public Health Reform and the Prevention of Infant Mortality, 1850–1929*. Baltimore: Johns Hopkins Press.

Melchert, Dennis D. 1973. Experimenting on The Neighbors: Inoculation of Smallpox in Boston in the Context of Eighteenth Century Medicine. Ph.D. thesis, University of Iowa.

Meldrum, Marcia. 1994. "Departures from the Design": The Randomized Clinical Trial in Historical Context, 1846–1970. Ph.D. thesis, State University of New York, Stony Brook.

Mendelsohn, Robert S. 1979. *Confessions of a Medical Heretic*. Chicago: Contemporary Books.

———. 1981. *Mal[e]practice*. Chicago: Contemporary Books.

———. 1984. *How to Raise a Healthy Child . . . In Spite of Your Doctor*. New York: Ballentine Books.

Merz, Beverly. 1987. HIV Vaccine Approved for Clinical Trials. *JAMA 258*: 1433–34.

Meyer, Harry M. 1969. Panel Discussion on Future of Rubella Virus Vaccines. *American Journal of Diseases of Children 118*: 395.

Meyer, Harry M., P. D. Parkman, T. E. Hobbins, and F. A. Ennis. 1968. Clinical Studies with Experimental Live Rubella Virus Vaccine (Strain HPV-77). *American Journal of Diseases of Children 115* (June): 648–54.

Mill, John Stuart. 1884[1843]. *A System of Logic, Ratiocinative and*

Inductive, Being a Connected View of the Principles of Evidence and the Methods of Scientific Investigation. London: Longmans, Green, & Co.

Miller, Henry I. 2004. Flu Shot Shortage. *Newsday*, 12 October, p. A41.

Miller, Vera. 1940. A Sociological Study of the Diphtheria Antitoxin, Its Investigation, Its Introduction and Diffusion in the United States, and the Resistance to Its Adoption. Master's thesis, University of Chicago.

Miniño, Arialdi M., Melonie Heron, and Betty L. Smith. 2006. Deaths: Preliminary Data for 2004. *National Vital Statistics Report* 54, no. 15 (28 June).

Mitchell, Alison. 1997. Clinton Calls for AIDS Vaccine as Goal. *The New York Times*, 19 May, p. B8.

Moore, John, and Roy Anderson. 1994. The WHO and Why of HIV Vaccine Trials. *Nature* 372 (24 November): 313–14.

Morse, John Lovett. 1916. Whooping Cough; the Measures to be Taken for Its Control and Prevention. *Boston Medical and Surgical Journal* 175, 723–27.

Mosier, D. E., R. J. Gulizia, S. M. Baird, D. B. Wilson, D. H. Spector, and S. A. Spector. 1991. Human Immunodeficiency Virus Infection of Human-PBL-SCID Mice. *Science* 251, no. 4995 (15 February): 791–94.

Moulin, A. 1991. *Le Dernier Langage de la Medécine: Histoire de l'immunologie de Pasteur au Sida.* Paris: Presses Universitaires de France.

Murphy, Jane. 1993. *What Every Parent Should Know About Childhood Immunization.* Boston: Earth Healing Products.

Murray, Patricia Carmen. 1987. DTP Vaccine Related Injury: An Examination of Proposed Vaccine Injury Compensation Legislation. *Journal of Contemporary Health Law and Policy* 3 (Spring): 233–51.

Murray, Roderick. 1969. Biologic Control of Virus Vaccines. *American Journal of Diseases of Children* 118 (August) 334–37.

Murrow, Edward R., and Jonas E. Salk. 1955. *See It Now.* 12 April.

Muula, A. S. 2007. Male Circumcision to Prevent HIV Transmission and Acquisition: What Else Do We Need to Know? *AIDS and Behavior* 11, no. 3 (May): 357–63.

Nathanson, Neal. 1999. Department of Health and Human Services Statement on Fiscal Year 2000 President's Budget Request for the National Institutes of Health (*www.oar.nih.gov/public/testimo.htm*).

Nathanson, N., and A. D. Langmuir. 1963. The Cutter Incident. Poliomyelitis Following Formaldehyde Inactivated Poliovirus Vaccination in the United States During the Spring of 1955. II. Relationship of Poliomyelitis to Cutter Vaccine. *American Journal of Hygiene* 78: 29–60.

National Committee for the Protection of Human Subjects of Biomedical and Behavioral Research. 1978. *The Belmont Report: Ethical Principles and Guidelines for the Protection of Human Subjects of Research.* Washington, D.C.: U.S. Department of Health, Education, and Welfare.

National Institutes of Health. 2006. Estimates of Funding for Various Diseases, Conditions, Research Areas. Search website at *www.nih.gov.*

National Vaccine Information Center. 1998. About Us (*nvic.org/About.htm*).

National Vaccine Information Center/Dissatisfied Parents Together. 1993. They Had No Voice . . . They Had No Choice, pamphlet.

NCPHSBBR, *see* National Committee for the Protection of Human Subjects of Biomedical and Behavioral Research.

Neff, John M., and David H. Carver. 1970. Rubella Immunization: Reconsideration of Our Present Policy. *American Journal of Epidemiology* 92, no. 3: 162–63.

NEJM, *see New England Journal of Medicine.*

Nelkin, Dorothy. 1992. Science, Technology, and Political Conflict: Analyzing the Issues. In *Controversy: Politics of Technical Decisions*, 3d ed., edited by Dorothy Nelkin. Newbury Park, Calif.: Sage.

Nelson, M. C., and J. Rogers. 1992. The Right to Die? Anti-vaccination Activity and the 1874 Smallpox Epidemic in Stockholm. *Social History of Medicine* 5: 369–88.

Nesmith, Jeff, and M. A. J. McKenna. 2004. Election 2004: Partisan Furor Erupts Over Vaccine Issue. *Atlanta Journal-Constitution*, 27 October, p. A9.

Neustadt, Richard E., and Harvey V. Fineberg. 1983. *The Epidemic that Never Was: Policy Making and the Swine Flu Scare.* New York: Vintage Books.

Neustadter, Randall. 1990. *The Immunization Decision: A Guide for Parents.* Berkeley, Calif.: North Atlantic Books.

New England Journal of Medicine. 1952. Rubella in Pregnancy, Editorial. *New England Journal of Medicine* 247, no. 4: 132–33.

New York Times. 1920. End of Diphtheria Assured by Experts. 1 March, p. 8.

———. 1926. Preventing Diphtheria. 9 September, p. 22.

———. 1932. Diphtheria Toxoid Announced by Parran. 16 May, p. 18.

———. 1947. 2D Smallpox Death Spurs Vaccination. 13 April, p. 1ff.

———. 1963. Vaccine Search Is Pushed. 9 June, p. 6.

———. 1965a. The Ravages of Rubella. 25 April, p. E7.

———. 1965b. The Ravages of Rubella. 28 April, p. 44.

———. 1979. Vaccine Recalled After Deaths of 4 Babies. 22 March, p. 17.

———. 1982. Two Ounces of Prevention. 18 May, p. A22.

———. 1986. Letter to the Editor. 27 March, p. A26.

———. 2004. An Influenza Vaccine Debacle, Editorial. 20 October, p. A26.

NIH, *see* National Institutes of Health.

Norman, Colin. 1985a. Congress Readies AIDS Funds Transfusion. *Science* 230, no. 4720 (25 October): 418–19.

———. 1985b. AIDS Trends: Projections from Limited Data. *Science* 230, no. 4729 (29 November): 1018–21.

———. 1985c. Africa and the Origin of AIDS. *Science* 230, no. 4730 (6 December): 1141.

———. 1985d. AIDS Therapy: New Push for Clinical Trials. *Science* 230, no. 4732 (20 December): 1355–58.

————. 1985e. AIDS Virus Presents Moving Target. *Science* 230, no. 4733 (27 December): 1357.

————. 1986. An Avalanche of New Cash. *Science* 230, no. 4734 (3 January): 12.

Nowak, Rachel. 1995. A Model Collaboration Built to Last. *Science* 269, no. 5229 (8 September): 1333.

NVIC, *see* National Vaccine Information Center.

NVIC/DPT, *see* National Vaccine Information Center/Dissatisfied Parents Together.

NYT, *see New York Times*.

Orenstein, W. A., K. J. Bart, A. R. Hinman, S. R. Preblud, W. L. Greaves, S. W. Doster, C. Stetlr, and B. Sirotkin. 1984. The Opportunity and Obligation to Eliminate Rubella from the United States. *JAMA* 251: 1988–94.

Oski, Frank A. 1990. *Principles and Practice of Pediatrics*, 2d ed. Philadelphia: J. B. Lippincott Co.

Osmundsen, John A. 1965. A Blood Test is Devised for German Measles. *The New York Times*, 21 April, p. 27.

Palca, Joseph. 1990a. A Reliable Animal Model for AIDS. *Science* 248, no. 4959 (1 June): 1078.

————. 1990b. African AIDS: Whose Research Rules? *Science* 250, no. 4978 (12 October): 199–201.

————. 1991a. AIDS: The Evolution of an Infection. *Science* 254, no. 5034 (15 November): 941.

————. 1991b. NCI Collaborations Suspended. *Science* 251, no. 4999 (15 March): 1306.

————. 1992a. A Surprise Animal Model for AIDS. *Science* 256, no. 5064 (19 June): 1630–31.

————. 1992b. Errant HIV Strain Renders Test Virus Stock Useless. *Science* 256, no. 5062 (5 June): 1387–88.

————. 1992c. Testing Target Date Looms, But Will the Vaccines Be Ready? *Science* 257, no. 5076 (11 September): 1472–73.

————. 1992d. The Case of the Florida Dentist. *Science* 255, no. 5043 (24 January): 392–94.

Parish, H. J. 1965. *A History of Immunization*. Edinburgh: E. & S. Livingstone, Ltd.

Park, William H. 1913. Active Immunization in Diphtheria by Toxin-Antitoxin Mixture. *American Journal of Obstetrics* 68, 1213–15.

————. 1922a. A Comparison Between the Amount of Diphtheria Developing Among 90,000 Children Who Had Been Tested by the Schick Test and, If Positive, Injected with Toxin-Antitoxin and 90,000 Untreated Children. In *Transactions of the Association of American Physicians* 37: 426–29.

————. 1922b. Toxin-Antitoxin Immunization against Diphtheria. *JAMA* 79, no. 19 (4 November): 1584–91.

————. 1931. The History of Diphtheria in New York City. *American Journal of Diseases of Children* 62, no. 6 (December), 1439–45.

Park, William H., and Abraham Zingher. 1915. Active Immunization with Diphtheria Toxin-Antitoxin and with Toxin-Antitoxin Combined with Diphtheria Bacilli; Second Paper; Late Results. *JAMA* 65: 2216–20.

———. 1916. The Late Results Obtained in the Active Immunization with Mixtures of Diphtheria Toxin-Antitoxin and with Toxin-Antitoxin Combined with Diphtheria Bacilli. *Journal of Immunology* 1: 127.

Parkman, Paul D., E. L. Buescher, and M. S. Artenstein. 1962. Recovery of Rubella Virus From Army Recruits. *Proceedings of the Society for Experimental Biology and Medicine* 111: 225–30.

Paul, John R. 1971. *A History of Poliomyelitis*. New Haven, Conn.: Yale University Press.

Paul, Yash. 2004. Herd Immunity and Herd Protection. *Vaccine* 22, no. 3–4 (January): 301–2.

PCSEPMBBR, *see* President's Commission for the Study of Ethical Problems in Medicine and Biomedical and Behavioral Research.

Perkins, Frank T. 1969. Panel Discussion on Future of Rubella Virus Vaccines. *American Journal of Diseases of Children* 118 (August): 382–96.

Peters, O. H. 1907. The Limited Value of Diphtheria Antitoxin as a Prophylactic. *British Medical Journal* 2: 865–67.

Petit, Charles. 1986. California to Vote on AIDS Proposition. *Science* 234, no. 4774 (17 October): 277–78.

PHSACIP, *see* Public Health Service Advisory Committee on Immunization Practices.

Pickering, Larry K., ed. 2000. *Red Book: Report on the Committee of Infectious Diseases*. Elk Grove Village, Ill.: American Academy of Pediatrics.

Pierce, C. C. 1925. Some Reasons for Compulsory Vaccination. *The Boston Medical and Surgical Journal* 192, no. 15 (19 April): 689–95.

Pinkerton, Steve D., and Paul R. Abramson. 1993. A Magic Bullet against AIDS? *Science* 262, no. 5131 (8 October): 162–63.

Pipes, Sally. 2005. Let My Vaccines Go. *MarketPlace*, American Public Radio, 9 November.

Place, E. H. 1913. In "Discussion," following Active Immunization in Diphtheria by Toxin-Antitoxin Mixture, by William H. Park. *American Journal of Obstetrics* 68: 1213–15.

Plotkin, Stanley A., David Cornfield, and Theodore Ingalls. 1965. Studies of Immunization with Living Rubella Virus: Trials in Children with a Strain from an Aborted Fetus. *American Journal of Diseases of Children* 110 (October): 381–89.

Plotkin, Stanley A., and Walter A. Orenstein, eds. 2004. *Vaccines*, 4th ed. Philadelphia: Elsevier.

Pollack, Andrew. 2004. U.S. Will Miss Half Its Supply of Flu Vaccine. *The New York Times*, 6 October, p. A1.

———. 2007. In Need of a Booster Shot: Rising Costs Make Doctors Balk at Giving Vaccines. *The New York Times*, 24 March, p. C1.

Polletta, Francesca. 1998. Contending Stories: Narrative in Social Movements. *Qualitative Sociology* 21, no. 4 (winter): 419–46.

Pool, Ithiel De Sola. 1959. *Trends in Content Analysis.* Urbana: University of Illinois Press.

Porter, Dorothy, and Roy Porter. 1988. The Politics of Prevention: Anti-Vaccinationism and Public Health in Nineteenth Century England. *Medical History* 32: 231–52.

Porter, Roy. 1996. *Cambridge Illustrated History of Medicine.* New York: Cambridge University Press.

Preblud, Stephen R., Alan R. Hinman, and Kenneth L. Herrmann. 1980. An Evaluation of the United States' Rubella Immunization Program. *American Annals of the Deaf* 125: 968–76.

President's Commission for the Study of Ethical Problems in Medicine and Biomedical and Behavioral Research's. 1982. *Compensating for Research Injuries: The Ethical and Legal Implications of Programs to Redress Injured Subjects.* Washington, D.C.: Government Printing Office.

Prickett, Stephen. 2002. *Narrative, Religion and Science: Fundamentalism Versus Irony, 1700–1999.* Cambridge: Cambridge University Press.

Prinzie, Abel, Constant Huygelen, Jeremy Gold, J. Farquhar, and J. McKee. 1969. Experimental Live Attenuated Rubella Virus Vaccine. *American Journal of Diseases of Children* 118: 172-77.

Public Health Service Advisory Committee on Immunization Practices. 1969. Recommendation of the Public Health Services Advisory Committee on Immunization Practices. *American Journal of Diseases of Children* 118: 397–99.

———. 1971. Rubella Virus Vaccine: Recommendation of the Public Health Services Advisory Committee on Immunization Practices. *Annals of Internal Medicine* 75, no. 5: 757–59.

Purdy, J. S. 1907. Malignant Diphtheria and the Immunizing Power of Antitoxin. *JAMA* 48, no. 26 (29 June): 2184.

Putney, S. D., T. J. Matthews, W. G. Robey, D. L. Lynn, M. Robert-Guroff, W. T. Mueller, A. J. Langlois, J. Ghrayeb, S. R. Petteway Jr, and K. WeinholdJ. 1986. HTLV-III/LAV-Neutralizing Antibodies to an *E. coli*-Produced Fragment of the Virus Envelope. *Science* 234, no. 4782 (12 December): 1392–95.

Putney, Scott D. and Dani B. Bolognesi. 1990. *AIDS Vaccine Research and Clinical Trials.* New York: Marcel Decker.

Quinn, T. C., J. M. Mann, J. W. Curran, and P. Piot. 1986. AIDS in Africa: An Epidemiologic Paradigm. *Science* 234, no. 4779 (21 November): 955–63.

Rabin, Roni. 2006. A New Vaccine for Girls, But Should It Be Compulsory? *The New York Times,* 18 July, p. F5.

Radbil, Samuel X. 1943. Whooping Cough in Fact and Fantasy. *Bulletin of the History of Medicine* 13, no. 1 (January): 33–53.

Rawlings, I. D. 1910. The Campaign against Diphtheria and Scarlet Fever in Chicago. *JAMA* 55: 570–75, 578.

Razzell, P. E. 1977a. *The Conquest of Smallpox.* Firle, England: Caliban.

———. 1977b. *Edward Jenner's Cowpox Vaccine: The History of a Medical Myth.* Firle, England: Caliban.

Reynolds, Harry S. 1919. Fifty-one Cases of Pertussis Treated with Vaccines. *Archives of Pediatrics* 36: 290–92.

Riddle, John M. 1997. *Eve's Herbs: A History of Contraception and Abortion in the West.* Cambridge: Harvard University Press.

Riessman, Catherine Kohler. 2004. Narrative Analysis. In *Encyclopedia of Social Science Research Methods,* edited by M. S. Lewish-Beck, A. Bryman, and T. Futing Laio. Malden, Mass.: Blackwell Publishing.

Rigau-Pérez, José G. 1989. The Introduction of Smallpox Vaccine in 1803 and the Adoption of Immunization as a Government Function in Puerto Rico. *Hispanic American Historical Review* 69, no. 3: 393–423.

Rogers, Anne, and David Pilgrim. 1995. The Risk of Resistance: Perspectives on the Mass Childhood Immunisation Programme. In *Medicine, Health and Risk,* edited by Jonathan Gabe. Oxford: Blackwell Publishing.

Rogers, Naomi. 1992. *Dirt and Disease: Polio before FDR.* New Brunswick, N.J.: Rutgers University Press.

Rosen, George. 1964. The Bacteriological, Immunologic, and Chemo-therapeutic Period, 1875–1950. *Bulletin of the New York Academy of Medicine* 40: 483–94.

———. 1965. Patterns of Health Research in the United States. *Bulletin of the History of Medicine* 39, no. 3: 201–21.

Rosenberg, Charles E. 1979. The Therapeutic Revolution: Medicine, Meaning, and Social Change in Nineteenth-America. In *The Therapeutic Revolution: Medicine, Meaning, and Social Change in Nineteenth Century America,* edited by Morris Vogel and Charles E. Rosenberg.

———. 1992. Introduction. In *Framing Disease: Studies in Cultural History,* edited by Charles E. Rosenberg and Janet Golden. New Brunswick, N.J.: Rutgers University Press.

Rosenberg, Tina. 2007. A Real-World AIDS Vaccine. *The New York Times Magazine* (14 January): 15–16.

Rosenkrantz, Barbara Guttman. 1972. *Public Health and the State: Changing Views in Massachusetts, 1842–1936* Cambridge: Harvard University Press.

Rothman, David J. 1991. *Strangers at the Bedside: A History of How Law and Bioethics Transformed Medical Decision Making.* New York: Basic Books.

Rothman, David J., and Sheila M. Rothman. 1984. *The Willowbrook Wars.* New York: Harper & Row.

Royer, B. Franklin, Paul G. Westen, and Glen F. Clark. 1908. A Study of Phagocytosis in Diphtheria. *Journal of Medical Research* 18: 107–26.

Runciman, W. G. 1989. *Max Weber: Selections in Translation.* New York: Cambridge University Press.

Sabatier, Reneé. 1988. *Blaming Others: Prejudice, Race, and Worldwide AIDS.* Philadelphia: New Society Publishers.

Sabin, Albert B. 1969. Panel Discussion on Future of Rubella Virus Vaccines. *American Journal of Diseases of Children* 118: 382–96.

———. 1991. Effectiveness of AIDS Vaccines. *Science* 251, no. 4998 (8 March): 1161

Salk, Jonas, P. A. Bretscher, Peter Salk, M. Clerici, and G.M. Shearer. 1993. A Strategy for Prophylactic Vaccination against HIV. *Science* 260, no. 5112 (28 May): 1270–72.

Samuels, Suzanne Uttaro. 1995. *Fetal Rights, Women's Rights: Gender Equality in the Workplace.* Madison: University of Wisconsin Press.

Santoli, Jeanne M., Natalie J. Huet, Philip J. Smith, Lawrence E. Barker, Lance E. Rodewald, Moira Inkelas, Lynn M. Olson, and Neal Halfon. 2004. Insurance Status and Vaccination Coverage Among U.S. Preschool Children. *Pediatrics* 113: 1959–64.

Sauer, Lewis W. 1933a. Whooping Cough: A Study in Immunization. *JAMA* 100, no. 4 (28 January): 239–41.

———. 1933b. The Preparation of Bacillus Pertussis Vaccine for Immunization. *JAMA* 102, no. 18: 1471.

———. 1935. The Known and Unknown of Bacillus Pertussis Vaccine. *American Journal of Public Health* 25 (November): 1226–30.

———. 1937. Municipal Control of Whooping Cough. *JAMA* 109, no. 7 (14 August): 487–88.

———. 1939. Whooping Cough: New Phases of the Work on Immunization and Prophylaxis. *JAMA* 112, no. 4 (28 January): 305–8.

Sawicki, Jana. 1991. *Disciplining Foucault: Feminism, Power, and the Body.* New York: Routledge.

Schackleton, William W. 1906. The Prophylactic Use of Anti-diphtheritic Serum. *Lancet* 2: 722.

Schanberg, Sydney. 1964. German Measles at Epidemic Rate. *The New York Times*, 8 February, p. 25.

Schibuk, Margaret Danielle. 1986. The Search for Vaccinia. Ph.D. thesis, Harvard University.

Schiff, Gilbert M., Hugo D. Smith, Peter St. J. Dignan, and John L. Sever. 1965. Rubella: Studies on the Natural Disease. *American Journal of the Diseases of Children* 110 (October): 366–69.

Schlesinger, Mark. 2002. A Loss of Faith: The Sources of Reduced Political Legitimacy for the American Medical Profession. *Milbank Memorial Fund* 80, no. 2: 185–235.

Schoenbaum, Stephen D., James N. Hyde, Louis Bartoshesky, and Kathleen Crampton. 1976. Benefit-Cost Analysis of Rubella Vaccination Policy. *New England Journal of Medicine* 294, no. 6: 306–10.

Schowalter, R. P. 1930. Value of Vaccine in Prevention of Whooping Cough. *American Journal of Diseases of Children* 39, no. 3 (March): 544–48.

Schroeder, M. C. 1921. The Duration of the Immunity Conferred by the Use of Diphtheria Toxin-Antitoxin. *Archives of Pediatrics* 38: 368–72.

Schwartz, Robert, and Andrew Grubb. 1985. Why Britain Can't Afford Informed Consent. *Hastings Center Report* 15, no. 4 (August): 19–25.

Seyer, John L., K. B. Nelson, and M. R. Gilkson. 1965. Rubella Epidemic, 1964: Effect on 6,000 Pregnancies. *American Journal of Diseases of Children* 110: 395–407.

Shapin, Steven. 1992. Discipline and Bounding: The History and Sociology of Science as Seen Through the Externalism-Internalism Debate. *History of Science* 30: 347–55.

Shaw, Edward B. 1940. The Prevention of Pertussis by the Use of Bacterial Vaccines. *Journal of Pediatrics* 17 (September): 414–16.

———. 1982. Pertussis Vaccine: Still an Open Question? Letter to editor. *Pediatrics* 69, no. 3: 386–87.

Shilts, Randy. 1987. *And the Band Played On: Politics, People and the AIDS Epidemic.* New York: St. Martin's Press.

Shorr, E, Y. 1936. Prophylactic Pertussis Immunization. *Journal of Pediatrics* 8 (July) 49–55.

Shorter, Edward. 1987. *The Health Century.* New York: Doubleday.

Shortt, S. E. D. 1983. Physicians, Science, and Status: Issues in the Professionalization of Anglo-American Medicine in the Nineteenth Century. *Medical History* 27: 51–68.

Siegel, M., H. T. Furst, and N. S. Peress. 1966. Fetal Mortality in Maternal Rubella: Results of a Prospective Study from 1957–1964. *American Journal of Obstetrics and Gynecology* 96 (15 September): 252–53.

Sill, E. Mather. 1913a. The Vaccine Treatment of Whooping Cough. *American Journal of Diseases of Children* 5: 379–85.

———. 1913b. The Vaccine Treatment of Whooping Cough. *American Medicine,* 8: 440–42.

Silverstein, Arthur M. 1981. *Pure Politics and Impure Science: The Swine Flu Affair.* Baltimore: Johns Hopkins University Press.

Simonds, A. P. 1978. *Karl Mannheim's Sociology of Knowledge.* Oxford: Clarendon Press.

Simpson, R. E. Hope. 1940. Rubella and polyarthritis. *British Medical Journal* 1 (18 May): 830.

Singer-Brooks, Charlotte H. 1940. Pertussis Prophylaxis: A Controlled Study. *JAMA* 114 (May): 1734–40.

Smith, Jane S. 1990. *Patenting the Sun: Polio and the Salk Vaccine.* New York: William Morrow and Company.

Smith, Philip J., Susan Y. Chu, and Lawrence E. Barker. 2004. Children Who Have Received No Vaccines: Who Are They and Where Do They Live? *Pediatrics* 114: 187–95.

Smith, Theobald. 1907. The Degree and Duration of Passive Immunity to Diphtheria Toxin Transmitted by Immunized Female Guinea Pigs to Their Immediate Offspring. *Journal of Medical Research* 16: 359–79.

Sontag, Susan. 1989. *AIDS and Its Metaphors*. New York: Farrar, Strauss and Giroux.

Spector, Bert. 1980. The Great Salk Vaccine Mess. *The Antioch Review* 38, no. 3 (summer): 291–308.

Spector, Malcolm, and John I. Kitsuse. 1987. *Constructing Social Problems*. New York: Aldine de Gruyter.

Spock, Benjamin. 1971. *Baby and Child Care*. New York: E. P. Dutton.

Stafford, Jane. 1940. The New Vaccine for Measles. *Science* 92, no. 2396 (20 September): 10.

———. 1941. Anti-Measles Vaccine. *Science* 93, no. 2411 (14 March): 9.

Starr, Paul. 1982. *The Social Transformation of American Medicine*. New York: Basic Books.

Stein, Rob. 2004. After Flu Shot Crisis, Demand Dwindles: High Risk Groups Do without Vaccine. *Washington Post*, 17 December, p. A3.

Stern, Bernhard J. 1927. *Should We Be Vaccinated? A Survey of the Controversy and Its Historical and Scientific Aspects*. New York: Harper & Brothers Publishers.

Stewart, G. T. 1978. Pertussis Vaccine: The United Kingdom's Experience. In *International Symposium on Pertussis*, edited by Charles R. Manclark and James C. Hill, 262–78. Bethesda, Md.: Department of Health, Education, and Welfare, Public Health Service, National Institutes of Health.

Stine, Gerald J. 1993. *Acquires Immune Deficiency Syndrome: Biological, Medical, Social, and Legal Issues*. Englewood Cliffs, N.J.: Prentice Hall.

Stolberg, Sheryl Gay. 1998. Eyes Shut, Black America Is Being Ravaged by AIDS. *The New York Times*, June 19, pp. A1, A12.

Stone, Richard. 1993a. Another Reversal for the AIDS Vaccine Trial? *Science* 260: no. 5112 (28 May): 1227.

———. 1993b. Army to Test Only MicroGeneSys Vaccine. *Science* 261, no. 5123 (13 August): 819.

———. 1993c. The True Cost of a Free AIDS Vaccine. *Science* 261, no. 5125 (27 August): 1107.

———. 1993d. Congress Seeks Answer to $20 Million Question. *Science* 262, no. 5131 (18 October): 167.

———. 1993e. Congress on gp160 Vaccine. *Science* 262, no. 5133 (22 October): 495.

———. 1993f. Endgame for MicroGeneSys Vaccine Trial? *Science* 262, no. 5140 (10 December): 1635.

Stovall, W. D. 1916. The Control of Diphtheria Epidemics. *JAMA* 66: 804–6.

Stratton, Kathleen R., Cynthia J. Howe, and Richard B. Johnston, Jr., eds. 1994a. *Adverse Events Associated with Childhood Vaccines: Evidence Bearing on Causality*. Washington, D.C.: National Academy Press.

———. 1994b. *DPT Vaccine and Chronic Nervous System Dysfunction: A New Analysis*. Washington, D.C.: National Academy Press.

———. 1994c. *Research Strategies for Assessing Adverse Events Associated with Vaccines*. Washington, D.C.: National Academy Press.

Sun, Marjorie. 1986. Vaccine Compensation Proposals Abound on Capitol Hill. *Science* 233, no. 4762 (25 July): 415.

———. 1988. Part of AIDS Virus Is Patented. *Science* 239, no. 4843 (26 February): 970.

Swan, Charles, A. L. Tostevin, Brian Moore, Helen Mayo, and G. H. Barham Black. Congenital Defects in Infants Following Infectious Diseases During Pregnancy. *Medical Journal of Australia* 2: 201–10.

Szasz, Thomas S., and Marc H. Hollander. 1956. The Basic Models of the Doctor-Patient Relationship. *Archives of Internal Medicine* 97: 585–92.

Szreter, Simon. 1988. The Importance of Social Intervention in Britain's Mortality Decline c.1850–1914: A Reinterpretation of the Role of Public Health. *Social History of Medicine* 1, no. 1 (April): 1–38.

Tenney, B. 1952. Progress in Obstetrics. *New England Journal of Medicine* 246, no. 16: 613–19.

Theiler, M, and H. H. Smith. 1937. The Use of Yellow Fever Virus Modified by In Vitro Cultivation for Human Immunization. *Journal of Experimental Medicine* 65: 787.

Thomas, Lewis, and Robert O. Marston. 1969. Welcome to Participants. *American Journal of Diseases of Children* 118, no. 1: 3, 5.

Thomas, Patricia. 2001. *Big Shot: Passion, Politics, and the Struggle for an AIDS Vaccine.* New York: Public Affairs Press.

Thomas, Stephen. B., and Sandra Crouse Quinn. 1987. The Tuskegee Syphilis Study, 1932–1972: Implications for HIV Education and AIDS Risk Education Programs in the Black Community. *American Journal of Public Health* 81, no. 11 (November): 1498–1505.

Thompson, Lea. 2000. Personal communication to the author, 2 October.

Thompson, Lea, and David Nuell. 1982. DPT: Vaccine Roulette. Washington, D.C.: WRC-TV (NBC). Video recording.

Thompson, Tommy. 2004. Quoted in Ask the White House, 19 October (*www. whitehouse.gov/ask/20041019-2.html*).

Thomson, William A. R. 1969. *Black's Medical Dictionary*, 28th ed. New York: Barnes & Noble.

Thurber, James. 1957. Here Lies Miss Groby. In *The Thurber Carnival*. New York: Modern Library.

Thursfield, J. Hugh. 1909. Pertussis or Whooping Cough. *Practitioner* 83: 487–500.

Tilly, Charles. 1984. *Big Structures, Large Processes, Huge Comparisons.* New York: Russel Sage Foundation.

Times of London. 1979. *Suffer the Children: The Story of Thalidomide.* New York: Viking.

Tingle, A. J., L. A. Mitchell, M. Grace, P. Middleton, R. Mathias, L. MacWillian, and A. Chalmers. 1997. Randomized Double-Blind Placebo-Controlled Study on Adverse Effects of Rubella Immunisation in Seronegative Women. *Lancet* 349 (3 May): 1277–81.

Tomes, Nancy. 1998. *The Gospel of Germs*. Cambridge: Harvard University Press.

———. 2001. Merchants of Health: Medicine and Consumer Culture in the United States, 1900–1940. *Journal of American History* 88, no. 2 : 519–87.

Tuller, David. 2006. Scientists Testing Vaccines to Help Smokers Quit. *The New York Times*, 4 July.

Uribarri, Adrian G. 2007. Proposal to Require HPV Vaccine Stirs Concerns. *Los Angeles Times*, 12 February, p. B3.

U.S. Vital Statistics. 1975. *Historical Statistics of the United States: Colonial times to 1970*. Washington, D.C.: U.S. Department of Commerce.

Veale, H. 1866. History of Epidemic Rothlen with Observations on its Pathology. *Edinburgh Medical Journal* 12: 404–14. Quoted in Preblud, Stephen R., Alan R. Hinman, and Kenneth L. Herrmann. 1980. An Evaluation of the United States' Rubella Immunization Program. *American Annals of the Deaf* 125: 968–76.

Veeder, Borden S. 1914. Active Immunization against Diphtheria by Means of von Behring's Vaccine and the Diphtheria Toxin Skin Reaction. *American Journal of Diseases of Children* 8: 154–62.

Vogel, Morris J., and Charles Rosenberg, eds. 1979. *The Therapeutic Revolution: Medicine, Meaning, and Social Change in Nineteenth Century America*. Philadelphia: University of Pennsylvania Press.

Volberding, Paul, and Donald Abrams. 1985. Clinical Care and Research in AIDS. *Hastings Center Report* (Special Supplement, AIDS: The Emerging Ethical Dilemmas) 15, no. 4 (August): 16–18.

Von König, C. H. 2005. Use of Antibiotics in the Treatment and Prevention of Pertussis. *Pediatric Infectious Disease Journal* 24, no. 5: S66-S68.

Von Sholly, Anna I., Julian Blum, and Luella Smith. 1917. The Therapeutic Value of Pertussis Vaccine in Whooping Cough. *JAMA* 68: 1451–56.

Wain, Harry. 1970. *A History of Preventive Medicine*. Springfield, Ill.: Charles C. Thomas.

Walgate, Robert. 2003. AIDSVAX Trial Not the End of the Story. *The Scientist* (28 February). Search at the-scientist.com.

Walters, LeRoy. 1988. Ethical Issues in the Prevention and Treatment of HIV Infection and AIDS. *Science* 239, no. 4840 (5 February): 597–603.

Warner, John Harley. 1992. The Rise and Fall of Professional Mystery: Epistemology, Authority, and the Emergence of Laboratory Medicine in Nineteenth Century America. In *The Laboratory Revolution in Medicine*, edited by Andrew Cunningham and Perry Williams, 110–41. Cambridge: Cambridge University Press.

Watters, John K. 1996. Americans and Syringe Exchange: Roots of Resistance. In *AIDS, Drugs, and Prevention: Perspectives on Individual and Community Action*, edited by Tim Rhodes and Richard Hartnoll, 22–41. New York: Routledge.

Weibel, Robert E., J. Stokes, Jr., Eugene Buynak, and M. R. Hilleman.

1969. Live Rubella Vaccine in Adults and Children. *American Journal of Diseases of Children* 118: 226.

Weller, Thomas H. 1965. The Rubella Symposium. *American Journal of Diseases of Children* 110 (October): 347.

Weller Thomas H., and F. A. Neva. 1962. Propagation in Tissue Culture of Cytopathic Agents from Patients with Rubella-like Illness. *Proceedings of the Society for Experimental Biology and Medicine* 111: 215–25.

Wesselhoff, Conrad. 1947. Rubella (German measles). *New England Journal of Medicine* 236, no. 25: 943–50.

Willems, J. S., and C. R. Sanders. 1981. Cost-Effectiveness and Cost Benefit Analysis of Vaccines. *Journal of Infectious Diseases* 144: 486–93.

Williams, Kathi. 2000. Personal communication to the author (July 20).

Williams, Naomi. 1994. Implementation of Compulsory Health Legislation. *Journal of Historical Geography* 20, no. 4 (October): 396–412.

Wilsford, David. 1994. Path Dependency, or Why History Makes It Difficult but Not Impossible to Reform Health Care Systems in a Big Way. *Journal of Public Policy* 14, no. 3: 251–83.

Wilson, Graham S. 1967. *The Hazards of Immunization*. London: University of London, The Athlone Press (Heath Clark lectures).

Wilson, Samuel M. 1913. Whooping Cough; Its Treatment with a Vaccine. *New York Medical Journal* 2: 823–24.

Witte, John J., Adolf W. Karchmer, George Case, Kenneth L. Herrmann, Elias Abrutyn, Ira Kassanoff, and John S. Neill. 1969. Epidemiology of Rubella. *American Journal of Diseases of Children* 118: 107–11.

Wohl, Stanley. 1984. *The Medical Industrial Complex*. New York: Harmony Books.

Wollstein, Martha. 1909. The Bordet-Gengou Bacillus of Pertussis. *Journal of Experimental Medicine* 11: 41–54.

Woolgar, Steve, and Dorothy Pawluch. 1985. Ontological Gerrymandering: The Anatomy of Social Problems Explanations. *Social Problems* 32: 214–27.

Worboys, Michael. 1992. Vaccine Therapy and Laboratory Medicine in Edwardian England. In *Medical Innovation in Historical Perspective*, edited by John V. Pickstone, 84–103. New York: St. Martin's Press.

Zagury, Daniel, J. Bernard, J. Leibowitch, B. Safai, J. E. Groopman, M. Feldman, M. G. Sarngadharan, and R. C. Gallo. 1984. HTLV-III in Cells Cultured from Semen of Two Patients with AIDS. *Science* 226, no. 4673 (26 October): 449–51.

Zarembo, Alan. 2005. TV Ads for Drugs Help Boost Prescriptions, Researchers Say. *The Los Angeles Times*, 27 April: A10.

Zimmerman, R. K., S. R. Kimmel, and J. M. Trauth. 1996. An Update on Vaccine Safety. *American Family Physician* 54, no. 1 (July): 185–93.

Zingher, Abraham. 1917. Preparation and Method of Using Toxin-Antitoxin Mixtures for Active Immunization against Diphtheria. *Journal of Infectious Disease* 21: 493–96.

———. 1918. The Active Immunization of Children under Eighteen Months of Age with Diphtheria Toxin-Antitoxin. *Archives of Pediatrics* 35: 489–94.

———. 1920–21. Practical Applications and Uses of the Schick Test. *Journal of Laboratory and Clinical Medicine* 52: 117–23.

———. 1921. Diphtheria Preventive Work in the Public Schools of New York City. *Archives of Pediatrics* 38: 336–59.

———. 1922. Results of Active Immunization with Diphtheria Toxin-Antitoxin in the Public Schools of New York City (Manhattan and the Bronx). *JAMA* 78: 1945–52.

Ziporyn, Terra Diane. 1988. *Disease in the Popular American Press: The Case of Diphtheria, Typhoid Fever, and Syphilis, 1870–1920*. New York: Greenwood Press.

Index